D0934726

THE PSYCHOLOGY OF ULTIMATE CONCERNS

The Psychology of Ultimate Concerns

Motivation and Spirituality in Personality

ROBERT A. EMMONS

THE GUILFORD PRESS
New York London

© 1999 The Guilford Press
A Division of Guilford Publications, Inc.
72 Spring Street, New York, NY 10012
http://www.guilford.com

Printed in the United States of America

This book is printed on acid-free paper.

Last digit is print number: 9 8 7 6 5 4 3 2 1

Library of Congress Cataloging-in-Publication Data

Emmons, Robert A.
    The psychology of ultimate concerns : motivation and spirituality
in personality / Robert A. Emmons.
        p.   cm.
    Includes bibliographical references and index.
    ISBN 1-57230-456-1 (hc)
    1. Goal (Psychology)   2. Self-actualization (Psychology)
3. Happiness.   4. Motivation (Psychology)   5. Personality.
6. Personality—Religious aspects.   I. Title.
BF505.G6E58   1999
155.2′5—dc21   99-26409
                                                          CIP

For Yvonne and Adam

About the Author

Robert A. Emmons, PhD, Professor of Psychology at the University of California, Davis, received his doctorate in Personality and Social Ecology from the University of Illinois at Urbana–Champaign. He is a member of the American Psychological Association's Division 36 (Psychology of Religion), the Society for the Scientific Study of Religion, the American Academy of Religion, and a Fellow of the International Society for Quality of Life Studies. Professor Emmons is a consulting editor for the *Journal of Personality and Social Psychology* and the *International Journal for the Psychology of Religion*, and was formerly on the editorial board of the *Journal of Personality*. His research focuses on personal goals, spirituality, and subjective well-being, and he has received research funding from the National Institute of Mental Health, the John M. Templeton Foundation, and the National Institute for Disability Research and Rehabilitation (U.S. Department of Education).

Acknowledgments

I used to think that golf was the ultimate humbling activity. When I put away my golf clubs and began to write this book, I realized that I had been badly mistaken. Writing is the ultimate humbler. For a goals researcher, a book shouldn't be all that hard to write; to accomplish a major task, you simply have to break the large goal down into manageable subgoals and protect them from competing intentions. Unfortunately, I found that there was a considerable gap between theory and practice.

Nevertheless, the book was ultimately completed, but it would not have been without the help of numerous individuals that I wish to acknowledge. First, the research reported in this book was conducted with the assistance of undergraduate, graduate, and postdoctoral researchers with whom I've had the privilege of working. These include Laura King, Patricia Colby, Heather Kaiser, and Ken Sheldon at the graduate level; Myriam Mongrain and Cheryl Crumpler at the postdoctoral level; and undergraduates Matthew Dank, Chi Cheung, Emily Stemmerich, Tim Gomersall, and Keivan Tehrani, who all made especially significant contributions to the research and ideas contained here. Laura King, in particular, played a pivotal role in the early studies on personal strivings and well-being, and I am deeply grateful for her collaboration and friendship over the years.

A special thanks is owed to Ed Diener for his support and mentoring in graduate school and beyond. Professors from my undergraduate days who shaped my interests in psychology were Estelita Saldanha and William Gayton at the University of Southern Maine. A number of friends and colleagues have served as sources of information and inspiration over the years, and I have learned much from them, most notably Mike McCullough, Jefferson Singer, Dan McAdams, Eric Klinger, Ray Paloutzian, Jamie Pennebaker, Joel Aronoff, Paul Karoly, Larry Pervin, Brian Little, and Katariina Salmela-Aro. I am indebted to Rick

Levenson and Ken Pargament, who read the entire manuscript and provided extensive and constructive comments. Seymour Epstein, Warren Brown, Bruce Smith, and Stacey Anderson also read and commented on portions of the book.

I want to express a special note of thanks to Glen Snyder. I have profited greatly from my friendship with Glen over the last several years. His life exemplifies many of the principles contained in this book: purpose, direction, commitment, and spiritual intelligence. I thank Glen for knowing what really matters in life and for his passion in communicating it.

At the institutional level, I am grateful to the University of California, Davis, for generously providing resources and a pleasant working environment. I thank the John M. Templeton Foundation, whose funding supported the latter part of this project.

At The Guilford Press, I am grateful to the Editor-in-Chief, Seymour Weingarten, for patiently enduring missed deadline after missed deadline with nothing more than an occasional gentle query of "How's the book coming?" I also thank Anna Nelson for her painstaking work in the production process and Christine Luberto and Katherine Lieber for their marketing expertise.

Most of all, I am blessed by a loving and supportive wife, Yvonne, and son, Adam. Thank you, Adam, for not learning to crawl until Daddy was finished with the book. It is dedicated to both of you.

Contents

PART I

*Personal Goals:
An Approach to Personality
and Subjective Well-Being*

CHAPTER ONE

Introduction:
Motivation and Spirituality
in Personality

What makes life meaningful, valuable, and purposeful? How do people invest their lives with a sense of the significant? Of all of the goals that people strive for, which really matter? Since the mid-1980s I have attempted to derive scientifically based answers to questions such as these. I initiated a program of research that broadly defined, was designed to examine the link between motivational aspects of personality and psychological or subjective well-being. More specifically, my driving concern has been to understand how personal goals are related to long-term levels of happiness and life satisfaction, and how ultimately to use this knowledge in a way that might optimize human well-being. To address this question, I put forth an approach to personality and subjective well-being centering on the construct of "personal strivings": individualized goals representing the typical or characteristic objectives that individuals try to accomplish in their everyday behavior (Emmons, 1986).

This book is about goals. There is perhaps no characteristic more fundamentally human than the capacity to imagine future outcomes and to devise means to attain these outcomes. Psychology has recently rediscovered goals as theoretical constructs, as evidenced by a number of major volumes on goals and human behavior that have been published since the mid-1980s (Gollwitzer & Bargh, 1996; Cantor & Kihlstrom, 1987; Carver & Scheier, 1998; Ford, 1992; Frese & Sabini, 1985; Martin & Tesser, 1996; Pervin, 1989). These volumes summarize the substantial advances that have been made in the scientific understanding of human beings as active, intentional, goal-directed agents. In both basic and applied research, spanning cognitive to clinical psychology, knowl-

3

edge of the structural, process, and content aspects of goals has been rapidly accruing. In my own field, personality psychology, a major trend has become the representation of personality in terms of dynamic processes, emphasizing how individuals strive for personally defined goals, construe daily opportunities for the realization of these goals, and regulate their behavior in an attempt to progress toward that which is personally meaningful and self-defining. Goals provide a sense of meaning and purpose in life; without goals, it is difficult to imagine how one could lead a life that is meaningful and valuable.

My particular focus has been in articulating which aspects of goals promote optimal psychological well-being. This book, then, is also about happiness, or psychological well-being. In the 1980s and 1990s, scientific studies on happiness skyrocketed. Long ignored in professional psychological discourse, scholarship on the science of happiness has been gaining ground on the multitude of studies devoted to psychological distress. Scientists, clinicians, policy makers and the public now have at their disposal an unprecedented data base for making decisions concerning the quality of life of individuals and societies. There is ample evidence that people's conscious values and goals are potent contributors to their overall levels of happiness. To paraphrase Csikszentmihalyi (1990), goals and concerns determine the contents of consciousness, and hence the quality of our lives. Goals and happiness are inextricably linked: For many people, the primary goal in life is to be happy.

Goal attainment can be a benchmark for well-being. For example, Lawton (1996) defined psychological well-being as "the self-evaluated level of the person's competence and the self, weighted in terms of the person's hierarchy of goals" (p. 328). Yet happiness involves much more than simply arriving at one's goal, in fact, contrary to popular belief, goal attainment rarely leads to long-term happiness. The picture is more complicated than that, and has led researchers to pursue a number of fascinating questions. For example, is the mere possession of personally meaningful goals more important than their attainment? Is the anticipated pleasure of attaining a goal a stronger incentive than its actual realization? When it comes to happiness, are all goals created equally? Or are some goals more than others likely to facilitate the attainment of long-term happiness? Similarly, not all goals are equally meaningful. What determines the meaningfulness of a goal? I have summarized the research on personal goals and well-being in a number of empirical papers and review chapters in edited volumes (Emmons, 1986, 1989, 1991, 1992, 1996). This book is more than just a restatement of this research; it places earlier work within an overall framework of how goals make life meaningful, valuable, and worth living, and the role that spirituality and religion play in the investment of personal goals with significance.

This book is thus also about spirituality, or personal religiousness. Spirituality is on the rise, both culturally and scientifically. The United States, in particular, for some time now has been depicted in the media as a land where the search for the sacred is increasing in intensity as this century draws to a close. Best-seller lists overflow with titles reflecting spiritual concerns, popular television programs focus on the divine, and even the scientific study of religious and spiritual phenomena is enjoying a renaissance. A heightened sensitivity to spiritual concerns has become one of the defining characteristics of modern culture (Inglehart, 1990; Roof, 1993). Although historical generalizations can be risky, it appears that more than at any previous time in history, people are concerned with determining their place within an evolving universe (Ramachandran & Blakeslee, 1998). Embedding one's finite life within a grander all-encompassing narrative appears to be a universal human need, as the inability to do so leads to despair and self-destructive behavior (Singer, 1997). According to data recently published by the Princeton Religious Research Center, the percentage of Americans who believe that the influence of religion is increasing its influence (for better or worse) in society is now the highest it has been in 12 years ("Dramatic Rise Seen," 1998).

Spirituality, as typically defined in common parlance, is thought to encompass a search for meaning, for unity, for connectedness, for transcendence, and for the highest of human potential. Such an all-encompassing approach to spirituality may not be particularly useful for conducting scientific research on the topic and for achieving progress in the scientific understanding of it. Thus, one purpose of this book is to present an empirical approach to spirituality that does not trivialize or oversimplify some of the most profound sources of human striving.

It has become fashionable to make distinctions between what is spiritual and what is religious. Religion is a (more or less) organized search for the spiritual associated with a covenant faith community with narratives that enhance the search for the sacred. Various fields of psychology, in particular the more applied areas of clinical, counseling, health, and rehabilitative psychology, are becoming increasingly aware of and impressed by the centrality of religious and spiritual concerns in people's lives. Research is demonstrating the generally beneficial impact that these concerns have on psychological, physical, and interpersonal functioning (Kelly, 1995; Koenig, 1998; Martin & Carlson, 1988; Pargament, 1997; Richards & Bergin, 1997; Shafranske, 1996).

There is a robust connection between personal well-being and a concern with the spiritual. The "faith factor" emerges as a significant contributor to quality-of-life indicators such as life satisfaction, happiness, self-esteem, hope and optimism, and meaning in life. In a leading quality-of-life journal, Poloma and Pendleton (1990) concluded their review of the literature with the observation that "the concept of religion obviously is a domain that merits the serious study of those who research well-being" (p. 270). The link between faith and happiness has historically been a controversial one, for, beginning with Freud, psychologists have been known for their antipathy toward organized forms of religion. In no one has this disdain for religion been more evident than in Albert Ellis (1980), who is on record as stating that "devout and orthodox religiosity is in many respects equivalent to irrational thinking and emotional disturbance . . . the elegant therapeutic solution to emotional problems is to be quite unreligious . . . the less religious they are, the more emotionally healthy they will be" (p. 637). Examination of the theoretical and empirical literature, however, reveals opposing positions as well, including this comment almost a century earlier from William James (1902), regarded by most as author of the classic work in the psychology of religion: "Happiness! Happiness! religion is one of the ways in which men gain that gift. Easily, permanently, and successfully, it often transforms the most intolerable misery into the profoundest and most enduring happiness" (p. 146).

ULTIMATE CONCERNS IN PSYCHOLOGY

The central theme of this book can be summed up using a concept that was coined by the existential theologian Paul Tillich in the 1950s. In his classic analysis of the affective and cognitive bases of faith, Tillich (1957) contended that the essence of religion, in the broadest and most inclusive sense, is *ultimate concern*. Faith, according to Tillich, is the state of being ultimately concerned, that is, focused on concerns that have a sense of urgency unparalleled in human motivation. Ultimate concern is "a passion for the infinite" (1957, p. 8). Religion "is the state of being grasped by an ultimate concern, a concern which qualifies all other concerns as preliminary and which itself contains the answer to the question of the meaning of our life" (Tillich, 1963, p. 4). Although Tillich used the term "ultimate concern," I will use the plural "ultimate concerns" to refer to the multiple personal goals that a person might possess in striving toward the sacred. As we will explore in this volume, the concept of ultimate concern enables a bridge to be built from issues of ultimacy in the abstract to everyday concerns and goals where issues of ultimacy "meet the road."

Concerns over ultimate questions of meaning and existence, purpose and value, do find expression in one form or another through personal goals. In attempting to answer questions such as "Does life have any real meaning?" or "Is there any ultimate purpose to human existence?" individuals' implicit worldview beliefs give rise to goal concerns that reflect how they "walk with ultimacy" in daily life. In past research studies investigating personal goals, participants have reported the ultimate concerns of trying to "be aware of the spiritual meaningfulness of my life," "discern and follow God's will for my life," "bring my life in line with my beliefs," and "speak up on issues concerning people who have been wronged." The use of goal language in discussions of spirituality and religion may seem peculiar to those accustomed to dealing with issues of faith and belief. Yet there is a long history of viewing religious behavior as telic—as goal directed (Trout, 1931). One of the basic functions of a religious belief system and a religious worldview is to provide "an ultimate vision of what people should be striving for in their lives" (Pargament & Park, 1995, p. 15) and the strategies to reach those ends. In the second half of this book, I present an approach for identifying ultimate concerns through personalized goals and I demonstrate the relevance of these goals for understanding psychological well-being outcomes and personality integration. My objective is to examine the place of spirituality or personal religiousness within a motivational account of personality functioning. I contend that ultimate concerns should occupy a central place in the structure of personality.

Before we examine more closely the relationship between spirituality and personality, a word about *my* motivation. This book is not an apologetic for any particular religious or spiritual worldview. When I began my research program on goals, I had no professional interest in religious or spiritual issues. I was content to superimpose existing psychological categories onto what I was trying to understand. Yet because it is such a pervasive dimension of life, spirituality revealed itself repeatedly through the phenomena I was studying—personal goals, well-being, happiness, purpose, meaning, the psychology of possibility and human potential. Once I opened myself up to the possibility that meaningful information about human personality was being revealed through these channels, I realized that I could no longer afford the luxury of ignoring this information. To do so, I believe, would have been the equivalent of committing academic malpractice. As a personality psychologist who professed a desire to understand the person in his or her entirety, I was guilty of ignoring what for many people is precisely what makes their life meaningful, valuable, and purposeful. I was ignoring people's attempts to contact a deep and authentic source of striving, goals that come closer than any other, in defining who people say they are. The result of my "awakening" is the second half of this book. I should also add that in this book I take no formal position on the existence of spiritual realities. My concern is with the manifestation of the spiritual in people's lives through the goals they strive toward.

Through psychological research on motivation and well-being, a tremendous potential exists for progress to be made in understanding the spiritual side of personality. People are reverent of science yet hungry for real spirituality (McCullough, 1995). It has been suggested that as the nations of the world move into an era of postmaterialism in which sheer physical survival is no longer the major goal, well-being is likely to become a preeminent concern of societies throughout the world (Inglehart, 1990). As I write these words, Pope John Paul II is in the midst of a historic trip to communist Cuba, where he is urging Cubans not to flee their lands in search of material gains or a better life, but rather to focus on that which transcends time—spiritual values, commitments, responsibilities, relationships. Although materialist values became increasingly widespread with the rise of industrial society, there is reason to suspect that, ultimately, people will return to a renewed emphasis upon spiritual values (Inglehart, 1990). When other avenues fail to bring ultimate fulfillment, spiritual concerns rise in the value hierarchy in people's quest for a satisfying quality of life.

One of my goals in writing this book is to show that, as personality psychologists, we must take the religious side of life seriously, for failing to do so results in an impoverished scientific account of the person. In practical terms, omitting the spiritual prevents us from being able to fully account for outcomes central to human adaptation. A pair of distinguished clinical psychologists used even stronger language when they recently wrote, "If we omit spiritual realities from our account of human behavior, it won't matter much what we keep in, because we will have omitted the most fundamental aspect of human behavior" (Richards & Bergin, 1997, p. xi). It is my belief that the psychological sciences are on the verge of a spiritual revolution. There have never been as many opportunities to advance scientific research on spirituality as exist today. Philosophies of science are changing so as to acknowledge the existence of, or at least to admit serious discussion of, transcendent realities (Richards & Bergin, 1997). Research that documents the role of spirituality in personal and societal well-being will play a major role in this revolution. In order to advance theory on spirituality and well-being, we need a theologically informed model of personality, one that is rooted in both the world's great wisdom traditions as well as contemporary empirical research. As a step in that direction, this book, then, is an attempt to bridge the secular-to-sacred gap in contemporary personality psychology.

OVERVIEW OF THE BOOK

The first part of the book presents an approach to personality and subjective well-being through the lens of personal striving theory. Telic models of well-being (Diener, 1984) assume that happiness is a function of the status of one's goal pursuits; formulaic conceptions of happiness generally posit that well-being is a function of an attainment-to-aspiration ratio. Chapter 2 deals with personality and purpose: goals as units of analysis in personality psychology. The recent goals revolution in psychology, the place of goals within motivational functioning, and issues in the measurement of personal goal units are the primary topics of concern.

In Chapter 3, I present an overview of the research findings on personal goals and subjective well-being. I first examine the nature of well-being, conceptually and methodologically. How have researchers operationalized the concepts of happiness and life satisfaction? Goal approaches to well-being have become increasingly popular in recent years, and the balance of the chapter is devoted to a synthesis of the existing knowledge base. I employ a framework that considers three primary aspects of goals: content, orientation, and structure. The last section of the chapter is an application of goal principles to therapeutic contexts, in which some contributions of a goal framework for understanding clinical and health issues are detailed. Cognitive-behavioral perspectives on treatment emphasize skill acquisition and everyday problem solving; goals are workable clinical units that can enhance cognitive-behavioral interventions.

While many aspects of goals facilitate subjective well-being, not all are beneficial. Conflicting aspirations are a major cause of suboptimal well-being and can lead to self-regulatory failure. The research literature on goal conflict and well-being is described in Chapter 4. While conflict is often perceived of in a psychodynamic context as a largely unconscious process, recent research has demonstrated that conscious conflicts influence a variety of psychological and physical health outcomes.

The second part of the book, Chapters 5 through 8, expands and broadens the realm of goal influences on well-being to incorporate the spiritual and religious dimension of striving. In Chapter 5, I provide a rationale for and measurement strategy to assess "ultimate concerns"— spiritual and religious themes in personal goal strivings. After considering definitional issues of what constitutes spirituality and religion, I describe some of the advantages of a goal-based approach for conceptualizing and measuring spiritual motivation, and then present recent research on spiritual strivings and well-being. According to Tillich, ultimate concerns determine our being and our non-being; as we will see in this chapter, they also determine our well-being.

The next two chapters expand the scope of spirituality from its involvement in emotional well-being to its role in personality integration and personal meaning. Chapter 6 explores the link between religion and personality integration, where I advance the proposition that religion and spirituality can foster the integration or unification of personality. Theological and psychological perspectives on integration are discussed, and data bearing on the religion-as-integration hypothesis are presented. Chapter 7 deals with the issue of meaning. People need meaning to survive; religion provides a powerful source of meaning. Baumeister (1991) considered religion to be the "ultimate value base" (p. 196). The difference between a meaningful life and a happy life is addressed in this chapter, as is the role of personal goals as key elements in the meaning-making process.

In the concluding chapter, I sketch a developing framework for spirituality and personality that I call "spiritual intelligence." I describe the logic involved in conceiving of spirituality as an intelligence, and consider the evidence for it in light of contemporary models of intelligence. I conclude by considering the possibility that spiritual intelligence can serve as an integrative framework for motivation and spirituality within personality. More importantly, I contend that this framework can lead to a fundamental shift in how spirituality and religiousness are viewed within human functioning.

RELIGION AND PERSONALITY:
PAST AND PRESENT

This book is about religion and spirituality in the psychology of personality. In order to place this work in perspective, some background information is needed by way of a historical overview and a brief discussion of the current status of the relationship between the psychology of religion and personality psychology.

As recently as the late 1960s, the psychology of religion and the psychology of personality appeared to be lifeless fields of inquiry. Destined to become archaic relics nostalgically associated with psychology's past, researchers were discouraged from intellectual inquiry in what were perceived as terminal fields. In the opening sentence of a section titled "Religion and Personality Characteristics" in the chapter on religion in the *Handbook of Social Psychology,* Dittes (1968) stated, "it is a confession of the poverty and primitive state of this field to propose a section so grossly focused as the heading above indicates" (p. 636). The same year, Mischel (1968) published his devastating critique of psychodynamic and trait models of personality, leaving academic personality psychology reeling for the next two decades.

Interestingly, 30 years later, following the premature reports of their deaths, both the psychology of religion and the psychology of personality are experiencing something of a renaissance. Vigorous empirical and conceptual work is being carried out in both fields. A revival of personality psychology has been noted by several writers (Emmons, 1993; McAdams, 1996; Singer & Salovey, 1993), and the psychology of religion is similarly alive and well (Hill, in press; Paloutzian, 1996; Wulff, 1997). The field of personality emerged from the post-Mischelian age with a renewed vigor. To be sure, differences of opinion remain, but consensus has slowly emerged regarding answers to several of the most fundamental issues in the field, including the basic traits of personality, the genetic and evolutionary basis of personality differences, and the degree to which personality changes versus remains stable over time (Caprara, 1996; Heatherton & Weinberger, 1994; Loehlin, 1992). Two comprehensive handbooks of personality appeared in the 1990s (Pervin, 1990; Hogan, Johnson, & Briggs, 1997).

Scientific research into spiritual matters has increased as well and has not been limited only to what is normally seen as the purview of "religious psychology." Various fields of mainstream psychology, in particular the more applied areas of clinical and health psychology, are becoming increasingly aware of, and impressed by, the centrality of religious concerns in people's lives, as well as the impact that these concerns have on mental, physical, and interpersonal outcomes. Once considered a taboo topic, there now appears to be considerable momentum and interest building in the study of the psychospiritual component of people's lives. The psychology of religion as an identifiable subfield within the American Psychological Association (APA) has been growing rapidly within the past 25 years; a number of journals, textbooks, and edited volumes are witness to this trend (Paloutzian, 1996). A chapter on the psychology of religion has appeared for the first time in an introductory textbook (Santrock, 1997). Membership in APA's Division 36, the Psychology of Religion, has been on a steady incline.

Despite progress in each of these two subdisciplines of psychology, advances at the *convergence* of personality and religion have been unsystematic, scattered, and generally unintegrated within an overall organizational framework that could promote progress and stimulate theoretical and methodological advances. In comparison to its neighboring subdisciplines, contemporary academic personality psychology has lagged behind in acknowledging the spiritual side of the person. Unlike its more applied brethren, concerned with the alleviation of psychological suffering, the psychology of personality is typically concerned with matters less urgent. As I hope to demonstrate in this book, because of the pervasive influence of religion and spirituality on cognitive, emotional, and motivational functioning, personality psychologists cannot afford to ignore this realm of experience and be true to their subject matter.

The relative lack of attention to spiritual matters in mainstream personality psychology is surprising for two primary reasons. First, early pioneers in the psychology of religion, such as Gordon Allport (1950) and Gardner Murphy (1947), had their primary identity as personality psychologists. For contemporary researchers who identify themselves with the personological "study of lives" tradition, one would expect some interest in religious and spiritual issues. Though it was often regarded with suspicion, disdain, outright hostility, or a mixture of these, religion received considerable attention in Freudian, neo-Freudian, and other classical personality theories. Yet somewhere along the line, religion pulled a vanishing act from personality theory and from psychology more generally. Nearly half a century ago, Allport (1950) began his classic book on personality and religion by stating, "Among modern intellectuals—especially in the universities—the subject of religion seems to have gone into hiding. . . . The persistence of religion in the modern world appears as an embarrassment to the scholars of today. Even psychologists, to whom presumably nothing of human concern is alien, are likely to retire into themselves when the subject is broached" (p. 1). Allport would not have been surprised to learn that a volume devoted to celebrating the 50th anniversary of his textbook (Craik & Hogan, 1993) made no mention of his extensive writings on the central role of the religious sentiment within the structure of personality. In addition, two recent, comprehensive handbooks of personality (Hogan et al., 1997; Pervin, 1990) fail to include religion as a topic of inquiry. A lone reference that appears in one (Megargee, 1997) bemoans this very neglect of the topic. Nor does the *Handbook of Social Psychology* (Gilbert, Fiske, & Lindzey, 1997) devote any space whatsoever to religion and social behavior. Out of a total of over 3,000 pages in these three presumably comprehensive handbooks, less than 1 page discusses religious influences on personality and social behavior. Baumeister and Tice (1996) suggested that whereas at one time personality psychology humbly incorporated perspectives from the humanities and other social sciences, the field became increasingly insular and preoccupied with microissues and internal debate in the wake of Mischel's (1968) call for accountability.

Another perplexing aspect of the neglect of religion is that personality psychology has long claimed to be concerned with understanding the whole person, which has always been championed as the unit of scientific study (McAdams, 1997). From the personalistic tradition of William Stern (1938) to Henry Murray's (1938) personological inquiries into human lives, the unifying agency of personality has been the linchpin distinguishing personality studies from other subdisciplines of psychology. Spiritual or religious goals, beliefs, and practices are central to many people's lives, and are powerful influences on cognition, affect, motivation, and behavior. Therefore, it would seem that in order to know a person (McAdams, 1995), personality psychologists must know about the religious side of people's lives. Spiritual or religious goals, beliefs, and practices are not only a distinctive component of a person, for many *they are* the core of the personality. National polls repeatedly report that over 90% of Americans believe in God. In one survey, nearly three-quarters of those polled nationally reported that "My whole approach to life is based on my religion" (Bergin & Jensen, 1990, p. 4). Thus, for at least a substantial percentage of the population an acute sense of spirituality is likely to be central to their goals, values, and motives. Now would be a propitious time to examine the links between personality and religion, both in terms of what the study of personality can contribute to the scientific study of religion and also what possible insights into personality structure and functioning an acknowledgement of the religious side of life can offer.

Part of my motivation for writing a book of this nature is my strong conviction that there is much to be gained by an increased dialogue between personality psychology and the psychology of religion and spirituality. Taking as its subject matter the development, functioning, and degree of transformation of the person over time, personality psychology is ideally situated to stimulate progress in understanding religious and spiritual influences in people's lives. Personality psychology deals with fundamental questions of human nature, and indeed, theologies are psychological theories as well (Ingram, 1996; Spilka & Bridges, 1989). Personality theory and theology ought to be natural allies; both are concerned, ultimately, with what it means to be a human being. It has been argued that the academic discipline of theology can advance the understanding of humankind, "asserting human dignity, the value of each person, the worth of each individual; the value of society, of friendship, of human interaction; the importance of moral thoughts; the notion of responsibility and the hope of changing the negative aspects of life" (Foerst, 1996, p. 692).

A small number of professional training programs recognize and attempt to capitalize on the natural affinity between personality and theology. For example, Emory University's graduate Division of Religion offers doctoral studies in the "Theology and Personality Program," whose focus is the critical and constructive study of the person. One of the course groupings at the Pacific School of Religion in Berkeley, California, is entitled "Religion and the Personality Sciences," and consists primarily of course offerings in personality theory, pastoral counseling, and religious conversion. Garrett-Evangelical Theological Seminary at Northwestern University offers a specialization area of "Religion, Personality, and Culture" within their Master of Theological Studies program. Theologians have been more considerate of personality theory than personality theory has been of theology. Only one textbook in personality psychology (Cloninger, 1996) devotes as much as a few pages to discussing religious aspects of personality. Research-based textbooks may not be expected to devote much space to religious or spiritual processes as they are structured to document the dominant themes in the empirical literature. However, even theories of personality texts, at greater liberty to discuss broad conceptions of human nature, are for the most part similarly silent on religion (e.g., Monte, 1999). It would appear that, true to Allport's (1950) prophecy, religion is still in hiding.

Ignoring spirituality in personality theory and research will not make it disappear. Personality theory and research cannot take place in a theological black hole. To stay silent on spiritual matters is to take the position that they are unimportant for understanding individuality, although there is ample evidence to argue against this position. Religion and spirituality have more relevancy for personality than most personality psychologists are comfortable in admitting. Personality psychologists cannot afford to be parochial in outlook; the health and vitality of the discipline depends on interdisciplinary outreach (Baumeister & Tice, 1996).

I hope that this volume will stimulate and encourage personality psychologists to take a serious look at what insights into personality structure and functioning an acknowledgment of the religious side of life can offer. Over a half-century ago, Gardner Murphy (1947), toward the conclusion of his biosocial text on personality, boldly speculated:

> In a future psychology of personality there will surely be a place for directly grappling with the questions of man's response to the cosmos, his sense of unity with it, the nature of his aesthetic demands upon it, and his feelings of loneliness or of consummation in his contemplation of it . . . the response of man to his cosmos is a clue to him and to cosmos alike. . . . Our study of man must include the study of his response to the cosmos of which he is a reflection. (p. 919)

What a difference it could make if more contemporary personality psychologists had a vision as grand as Murphy's. This book is offered in the spirit of his inspiring challenge; I hope that in some small way it contributes to the agenda he envisioned.

CHAPTER Two

Personal Goals as Units of Analysis

*H*uman beings are by nature goal oriented. This is no longer a controversial truth claim in psychology, but neither is it a trivial one. The lives of human beings are structured around the pursuit of incentives—goals that we seek to obtain, maintain, or avoid. Survival of the individual, as well as of the species, is contingent upon the successful attainment of goal pursuits. It is not an overstatement to say that a goal revolution has occurred in psychology over the past 20 years. A goal-theoretical approach has become widely adopted by researchers in nearly every area of psychology, including social, personality, clinical, cognitive, developmental, evolutionary, organizational psychology, and the psychology of aging.

An examination of some recent positions makes the case for goals very clear. Developmentalists Ford and Nichols (1987) commented that individuals' "capacity for cognizing and pursuing goals is revealed in everyday experience . . . [and] is what gives meaning and purpose to people's lives" (p. 293). Karoly (1993), a cognitive-behavioral clinical psychologist, phrased it this way: "In the context of a resurgence of interest in purposiveness, self-direction, volitional control, and emotional modulation, the goal construct has been elevated to a preeminent status as a motivational variable" (p. 274). Lastly, in speculating on future trends in evolutionary psychology, Buss (1995) stated, "The next decade of psychological research should witness a sharp increase in attention paid to strategies, tactics, and goals as new units of analysis in personality psychology. The discovery of an underlying, species-typical goal structure will constitute a major and lasting scientific advance" (p. 21).

Austin and Vancouver (1996) provide a masterful review of the literature on goal constructs, from both an applied as well as from a basic

15

research perspective. Their review is organized around a structure, process, and content framework. Goal structure includes goal dimensions, properties, and organization; goal processes pertain to establishing, planning, striving, and revising goals; and goal content is the categorization of goals into taxonomies. They concluded their review with the following: "Whether one is interested in the key theoretical questions or the practical implications of psychology, the study of goal constructs promises to be a stimulating research area, particularly given their potential for integrating psychological domains" (p. 363).

But what exactly are goals, and what do they tell us about human personality? How have they been conceptualized within personality psychology? How can goals be measured in psychological research, and, in particular, in research bearing on goal theories of happiness, well-being, and optimal human functioning? These are the primary issues with which this and the next chapter are concerned.

Few would quarrel with the claim that human beings are goal directed. The definition of a goal is equally nonproblematic. Perhaps the most inclusive definition was provided by Austin and Vancouver (1996), who defined goals as "internal representations of desired states, where states are broadly construed as outcomes, events, or processes. Internally represented desired states range from biological set points for internal processes (e.g., body temperature) to complex cognitive depictions of desired outcomes . . . that span from the moment to a life span and from the neurological to the interpersonal" (p. 338). Individual investigators have placed their unique signature upon this generalized definition of a goal, and for research and applied purposes have developed a number of goal-related constructs. I review those formulations in a later section of this chapter.

GOAL STRIVING AS A BIOLOGICAL AND PSYCHOLOGICAL IMPERATIVE

Motivational constructs have returned to center stage in personality psychology partly due to the emergence of an evolutionary explanatory framework for personality processes (Buss, 1995; Klinger, 1998; MacDonald, 1995). Klinger (1998) has argued that goal striving is a fundamental feature of living organisms. Goals are life's basic ingredients, for without goals, life would cease to exist. Klinger has described this basic reality as "the imperative of purpose" and documents the core tendency of goal striving in all living systems. Human brains in particular, according to Klinger, are wired for purposeful living, and life itself is a virtual continuous stream of goal pursuits. The requirements of goal striving have the most pronounced effects on the direction that evolution will take. Accordingly, then, motivational systems are at the center of behavioral organization. Other systems, primarily the cognitive and affective, evolved in support of the motivational system. Thus, cognitive and affective processes have a specifiable set of functions that enable organisms to process environmental and internal information and to respond emotionally in ways that promote problem solving and goal attainment. It is easy to see why goals, according to Klinger (1998), serve as "the linchpin of psychological organization" (p. 44). Buss (1995) has argued for the importance of evolutionary goals such as mate acquisition, negotiating dominance hierarchies, forming reciprocal alliances, and other social goals of evolutionary significance. Buss is optimistic that an evolutionary analysis may yield insights into species-typical goal systems, that is, the powerful commonalities underlying the diversity of human striving.

GOALS WITHIN PERSONALITY PSYCHOLOGY

A complete understanding of the role of motivation and spirituality in personality requires an extended discussion of how personality is conceptualized by contemporary personality psychologists. Only then can the interplay between personality and religion, at both the level of theory and method, be effectively approached. Recent advances in the development of comprehensive frameworks for understanding the individual suggest that at least a minimal consensus may be achieved regarding the kinds of constructs to employ. Description of individuality is a fundamental goal of personality psychology; indeed, the history of personality psychology is a record of the search for appropriate units of analysis for studying the person. A bewildering array of possibilities awaits the contemporary personologist.

Personality psychology has had a dual nature throughout its 60-year history; these two sides of the discipline have been referred to as the "having" and "doing" of personality, or what personality "is" and what personality "does" (Cantor, 1990). Cantor (1990) traced the evolution of this dualism from the inception of the field in the 1930s to the present time. The identification of stable individual differences, representing the "building blocks" or basic structures of personality—what personality *is*—has been an objective of the field since its beginning. Recently, these efforts have come to fruition as psychologists have rallied around the five-factor model of personality (Wiggins, 1996). Five traits—openness to experience, conscientiousness, extraversion, agreeableness, and neuroticism (or OCEAN, for short)—offer a unifying frame of reference that seems to have been readily adopted by many inside and outside the field of personality psychology proper. The five-factor model has been bolstered by genetic studies of behavior demonstrating substantial heritabilities of many personality traits (Loehlin, 1992). The consensus of what personality "is" has become the traits identified by the five-factor model.

In contrast to the dispositional orientation, the cognitive-motivational approach to the person takes as its starting point what personality *does* rather than what personality *is*. Such an approach to the person is designed to elucidate the mechanisms by which the "having" side of personality is translated into concrete behavior sequences across situational and temporal contexts. A number of cognitive mechanisms are invoked to account for the translation of abstract dispositions into concrete action, including strategies, schemas, and tasks as well as personal strivings and goals.

FROM A TWO- TO THREE-LEVEL
MODEL OF PERSONALITY

McAdams (1996) recently articulated a framework for the understanding of human individuality. McAdams proposed that knowing a person requires being privy to information at three distinct levels or domains of personality description: (1) comparative dispositional traits, (2) contextualized personal concerns, and (3) integrative life stories. Each level contains different constructs and a different focus and is accessed through different measurement operations. The three levels are relatively orthogonal realms of functioning, unfolding independently of each other and differing in their accessibility to consciousness. They provide different vantage points or perspectives from which to approach the scientific study of persons, and to approach the study of motivation and spirituality within personality.

Level I is comprised of relatively nonconditional, decontextualized, and comparative dimensions of personality called "traits." Characteristics at this level are essential in describing the most general and observable aspects of a person's typical behavioral patterns. These essential ingredients of personality are global and enduring features of the person, what McCrae and Costa (1996) have referred to as "basic tendencies." As noted earlier, personality-trait psychology has recently culminated in what many have argued is a consensus around the five-factor, OCEAN, model of personality traits (Digman, 1990; McCrae & Costa, 1990). OCEAN has proven to be a powerful framework for organizing existing trait questionnaire measures and for predicting important life outcomes such as health and psychological well-being, and therapeutic outcomes.

Traits are valuable descriptive features of persons, owing to their normative and nonconditional properties. But people are not identical to their traits. To quote Ryan (1995), "Life is not lived as a trait" (p. 416). The limitations of decontextualized trait units for understanding individuality have been spelled out elsewhere (Block, 1995; McAdams, 1992; Pervin, 1994). Diener (1996) argued that while traits can account for considerable variance, they are insufficient for fully understanding the multiply-determined phenononmenon of subjective well-being. He demonstrates that trait constructs fail to offer a complete account of people's evaluative responses to their lives. McAdams (1992) argued that trait descriptions yield at best a "psychology of the stranger"; they are a preliminary attempt at describing a person.

Level II is comprised of contextualized strategies, plans, and concerns that enable a person to solve various life tasks and achieve personally important life goals. Recent years have seen an increasing articulation of constructs at this level of analysis as personologists turn their attention to self-regulatory mechanisms and structures that guide behavior purposefully to achieve desired goals. Constructs at this level, which include personal projects (B. R. Little, 1989), life tasks (Cantor, 1990), and personal strivings (Emmons, 1986) are characterized by intentionality and goal directedness, in comparison to the stylistic and habitual tendencies at Level I. Presumably more malleable than traits, these units are sometimes noncomparative, frequently highly contingent, and contextualized in time and space. Little (1996) refers to these units as Personal Action Constructs (PAC) and explicitly contrasts them with broad dispositions. Constructs at this level tend to be motivational and developmental in nature, focusing explicitly on what a person is consciously trying to do during a particular period in his or her life. They are "characteristic adaptations" (McCrae & Costa, 1996). As McAdams (1996) and Pervin (1994) have forcefully argued, concepts at this level are fundamentally different from traits and cannot be reduced to traits. Goals are not traits, nor are they genetically based to any significant degree (though there are few hard data on this). Karoly (1993) specifies the difference between goals and traits: "as something aspired to, a goal is inherently provisional, encompassing the romance of human possibilities—success, failure, frustration, disappointment, deferment, disallowance at the hands of others, and subversion by oneself" (p. 274).

Level III is identity or the life narrative. Identity is reflected in the stories that people construct to provide them with a sense of overall meaning and purpose to their lives. The life story renders the array of traits, strivings, and other various Level I and II elements into a more or less coherent and constantly evolving integrative unity. To quote Singer and Salovey (1993), "The stories individuals tell about their own lives are the life blood of personality" (p. 70). The "having" and "doing" sides of personality are encapsulated respectively in Levels I and II, whereas Level III is concerned with the "making" of the self (McAdams, 1996).

The three-level model of personality description offered by McAdams calls attention to the richness of personality and what elements are needed for a comprehensive understanding of the person. People *are* more than their traits. Although the three levels of description are depicted by McAdams as being relatively independent of each other, I suspect that this situation is for expository purposes. Within a concrete life, there is likely to be considerable interaction between features at the different levels. For example, a person may choose to work on his or her neuroticism (Level I) as a personal goal (Level II), with consequences for the telling of the life story (Level III). There is a need for research and theory into the dynamic links between traits, personal concerns, and life narratives. This integrative agenda for the field of personality psychology can stimulate advances in understanding links between personality processes and individual differences, and between idiographic and nomothetic levels of description. There is no reason why different aspects of personality functioning cannot ultimately be integrated within an overall viable theory of personality structure.

MOTIVATION IN PERSONALITY PSYCHOLOGY

Motivation has always been seen as central to personality psychology, although interest in motivational concepts has waxed and waned over the last 50 years. A concern with motivation and dynamics is one of the distinguishing features of the field. According to G. W. Allport (1937), "the problem of motivation is central to the psychological study of personality" (p. 196). Hogan (1976) argued forcefully that motivational concepts are the "explanatory concepts par excellence in personality psychology" (p. 50). Historically, concepts such as instinct, need, and drive carried the burden for motivational theorizing. As Pervin (1983) noted, though, the demise of drive theory in the late 1950s tended to result in a diminution of interest in motivational concepts in general. This was particularly disturbing as the pioneers in the field—Gordon Allport, Henry Murray, Ross Stagner, Kurt Lewin, David McClelland—all stressed the dynamic, striving character of behavior, that is, its movement toward largely idiosyncratic goals. For instance, of central interest to both Allport and Stagner was motivation. For G. W. Allport (1937), "Motivation is the go of personality, and is, therefore, our most central problem" (p. 218). According to G. W. Allport (1937), the intentions and motivational dispositions "tell us what sort of future a person is trying to bring about, and this is the most important question we can ask of any mortal" (p. 223). In addition, Allport notes, the unity of the self is reflected in goal-directed striving. Similarly, Stagner (1937) noted that "discussing personality without regard to dynamics (i.e., motivation) is like describing the exterior of an automobile . . . ignoring the characteristics of the engine" (p. 257). Both Allport and Stagner firmly believed in the idiographic basis of motivation. Allport championed the notion of personal dispositions, of which there were two types—stylistic and motivational. Stagner (1937) offered a cultural interpretation of motivation in which he argued that the motives toward which people strive are culturally determined, but also agreed that "to know completely the motivation of any personality, we must study that person" (p. 306).

The same year that G. W. Allport (1937) and Stagner (1937) were publishing their seminal texts, Gordon's older brother, Floyd Allport (1937), published an article in *Character and Personality* titled "Teleonomic Description in the Study of Personality." In this article, Floyd Allport proposed that personality traits were of limited utility for describing the personality of an individual. He suggested describing an individual's personality in terms of what the person seems to be "trying to do," or the purpose or purposes that he or she seems to be trying to carry out. Floyd Allport coined the term "teleonomic trend" to describe these behavioral tendencies, which he claimed were more dynamic and discriminating than trait terms, and he suggested that these teleonomic trends could be used to understand apparently inconsistent behavior (Pervin, 1983). For example, a child who is unruly and disruptive in the classroom might be well mannered and agreeable at home. These apparent inconsistencies at the behavioral level make sense at a deeper level by positing that the child is "trying to gain the attention of adults" and has learned flexible strategies for doing so in different environments. Unfortunately, the influence of the concept did not spread far from origination in Floyd Allport's work. A possible reason for this may have been the cumbersome method of assessing these trends, which required observer ratings from a large number of the person's associates. Floyd Allport did not believe that what an individual said about his or her motives should be taken at face value. There is reason, however, to believe that the concept was abandoned prematurely. The personal striving approach is heavily indebted to Floyd Allport and his pioneering work on teleonomic trends. Elsewhere I have described in detail the genesis of personal strivings within the teleonomic trend tradition (Emmons, 1989).

Following in the footsteps of the Allports, Murray, Stagner, McClelland, and other visionaries, theorists and researchers today are more willing to invoke motivational concepts into their descriptive and explanatory models. Terms such as tasks, goals, concerns, projects, strivings, and motives are part of the everyday motivational parlance. I (Emmons, 1997) have argued elsewhere that the recent revitalization of the field of personality that has occurred in the past two decades has been due in large part to a resurgence of interest in motivational concepts. Indeed, it has been suggested that we are in the midst of a "conative revolution" (Little, 1993). Both emotion and motivation, having long taken a back seat to behavior and cold cognitive approaches, are now at the forefront of much of our conceptual and empirical efforts.

Personality researchers are also addressing the interaction of units of personality at different levels of analysis. Addressing the relationship between motives and traits was the objective of Winter, John, Stewart, Klohnen, and Duncan (1998). Following a review of the history of the trait and motive distinction, the authors developed their "channeling hypothesis": that traits, as stylistic tendencies, channel or direct the ways in which motives, wishes, desires, and goals are expressed in particular actions and contexts throughout life. The indispensable, nonreducible role that each construct plays in predicting developmental outcomes was demonstrated in two longitudinal studies.

Goals as Motivational Units

During the 1980s there was increasing interest in using the goal construct to get a glimpse into human motivation. Within this framework, motivation is a key aspect of personality, as it lends direction, coherence, and pattern to behavior. Generally, motivation has been portrayed as the source of coherence in personality, as the force that brings meaning to apparent anomalies in behavior. Goals are part of a larger motivational system that forms a complex hierarchy, the levels of which differ in generality and abstractness of the intentions involved. Several successful research programs have made progress in uncovering the individual's goal structures, that is, his or her consciously articulated and personally meaningful objectives in life. Much of this work has been directed toward the identification of goal taxonomies and the development of individual differences in goal orientations, although other efforts have been aimed at uncovering individual construals of life goals (e.g., Cantor & Kihlstrom, 1987; Emmons, 1989; Ford & Nichols, 1987; B. R. Little, 1989). In spite of their differing objectives, these perspectives share the following assumptions:

1. Behavior is organized around the pursuit of goals, with goals being defined as objectives which a person strives to obtain or avoid.
2. Goals influence ongoing thought and emotional reactions in addition to behavior.
3. Goals exist within a system of hierarchically organized super-

ordinate and subordinate goals, where functioning in one aspect of the system has ramifications for other parts of the system.

4. Goals are accessible to conscious awareness, although there is no requirement that the goal be represented in consciousness while the person is in active pursuit of it.

Personal Goals

Among the goal units explored by personality psychologists in the 1980s and 1990s, consciously accessible, self-articulated personal goals have been proposed as the most optimal unit of analysis in motivational personality psychology. Rather than focusing on broad unconscious motives, researchers became interested in studying the mundane goals that drive daily behavior—the types of goals that a person might work on in his or her daily life. These personalized goal approaches provided a new way to look at motivation. For instance, these approaches assumed that the goals that drive behavior are available to awareness. In addition, these approaches acknowledged that in terms of daily life, motivational tendencies are constrained to a particular context. A number of personal goal constructs appeared on the psychological scene during this period, each with its range of convenience for explaining and predicting significant life outcomes such as subjective well-being. These include the constructs of current concerns (Klinger, 1977), life tasks (Cantor, 1990), personal projects (B. R. Little, 1989), personal strivings (Emmons, 1986), and personal goals (Brunstein, 1993).

In contrast to the broad traits or motive dispositions at Level I in McAdam's (1995) framework, personal goal constructs represent contextualized, circumscribed, and idiographic units that account for human motivation. They have been termed "middle-level" units of analysis for cognitive personality psychology in that they are typically at a middle level of abstraction in a structural hierarchy, and can be concretized with reference to specific activities and situations and generalized with reference to higher order themes and meanings in life. Each are ways of representing affectively charged goals and themes that are central to the person's life and that emerge from and determine the nature of the person's transactions with the social world. Cantor and Zirkel (1990) have eloquently argued that these middle-level units are cognitive in that they are organized around individuals' beliefs about themselves and their relationships, their autobiographies and identities, and their projects, tasks, and concerns that give meaning to life. These units are infused with motivational content and function as goals to energize and organize purposive behavior. Although each researcher invokes the concept of "goals," there are substantial differences in meaning, measurement, and hypothesized linkages within the personality.

Current Concerns

Eric Klinger (1977, 1998) has argued that experience is organized around the pursuit of incentives which are represented by a "current concern," or a hypothetical motivational state in between two points in time: the commitment to a goal and either the consummation of the goal or disengagement from it. This hypothetical state guides a person's ongoing thoughts, emotional reactions, and behavior during the time it is active. Klinger developed the notion of a "current concern" out of dissatisfaction with the failure of the broad motive dispositions to predict spontaneous thought content. However, Klinger does not posit the representation of the concern in consciousness; it is assumed that for the majority of the time, the concern is not reflected in on-line cognitive processing. People simultaneously possess a number of current concerns, as there is a different concern for each goal a person is committed to. The range of potential concerns is diverse, as each individual possesses an idiographic set which frequently changes. Examples of current concerns are "Finishing writing this book," "Planning a summer vacation in Maine," "Keeping a dentist appointment," "Losing weight," and "Maintaining a love relationship." Concerns may be defined narrowly or broadly, and may last anywhere from a few seconds to a lifetime.

Concerns are hypothetical nonconscious brain processes that keep a goal pursuit "psychologically alive" for a person and enable him or her to strive for goals and to resume goal striving following interruption of goal-directed activity. As controllers of conscious and unconscious mental content, concerns direct cognitive processing and demonstrate the dependence of consciousness on meaningful goals. In daily life, thoughts are triggered by environmental cues that are related to current concerns, and it is the emotional properties of concerns that affect the processing of these cues. Klinger's (1998) impressive research program has documented the ebb and flow of concerns in conscious mentation and in dream states. Amidst the rhetoric generated by the cognition and emotion debate in psychology, Klinger has provided a steady voice in elucidating the mechanisms of cognitive-emotional interactions in the processing of motive-relevant information.

Personal Projects

A similar though independently developed concept is the personal project (B. R. Little, 1989, 1993; McGregor & Little, 1998). Rooted in Murray's (1959) concept of a serial program, personal projects are "an interrelated sequence of actions intended to achieve a personal goal" (Palys & Little, 1983, p. 1223). Personal projects are things that people think about, plan for, carry out, and sometimes, but not always, complete. Everyday activity is organized around these personal projects. Examples of personal projects are "Going to the prom with Brad," "Finding a part-time job," and "Shopping for the holidays" (B. R. Little, 1989). The concept was developed and promoted by Little as an interactional unit that links the individual to his or her sociocultural context. Little (1993) stresses three types of contexts that are necessary for understanding action: the intentional context, in which the purposes underlying the projects are discerned; the systemic context, the relation of projects to each other within a project system; and the ecological context, the environmental and historical milieu in which the action takes place.

The personal project concept has proven effective in studies of subjective well-being. For instance, Palys and Little (1983) found that individuals who were involved in short-term important projects that were highly enjoyable and moderately difficult were more satisfied with their lives than individuals who possessed projects that were of longer range but from which they derived little immediate enjoyment. Ruehlman and Wolchik (1988) reported that interpersonal support and hindrance in personal project pursuit were related to well-being and distress, respectively, and that hindrance was also related to low well-being. Katariina Salmela-Aro (1992) at the University of Helsinki recently found that distressed Finnish college student clients seeking psychological counseling reported less success in project accomplishment and more projects related to self-focused concerns in comparison to two nondistressed groups.

Life Tasks

Nancy Cantor and her colleagues (Cantor, 1990; Cantor & Kihlstrom, 1987; Cantor & Zirkel, 1990) define life tasks as "the problem(s) that individuals see themselves as working on in a particular life period or life transition" (Cantor & Zirkel, p. 150). These life tasks, consensual in nature, organize and give meaning to a person's everyday activities, and are especially salient during developmental periods such as marriage or graduation from college. The life-task concept emerged within Cantor and Kihlstrom's (1987) social-cognitive approach to personality, an approach emphasizing discriminativeness, flexibility, and goals as knowledge structures facilitating problem solving in everyday life contexts. The life-task construct was originally developed in order to explore how people use social intelligence in dealing with tasks posed by life transitions. Examples of life tasks include "Succeeding academically," "Making friends," and "Being on my own." Whereas much of the personal goals research has examined goal appraisals across domains, Cantor and her colleagues have focused on goal appraisals in specific life domains, such as independence, intimacy, and achievement. Research on life tasks has been aimed at demonstrating how the cognitive basis (social intelligence) of personality is revealed in the problem-solving strategies chosen by the individual in approaching his or her life tasks. Cantor's seminal work on the cognitive basis of personality plays a pivotal role in the integrative framework of motivation, spirituality, and intelligence that I establish in the final chapter of this book.

Personal Strivings

Gordon Allport (1955) stated that "when we set out to study a person's motives, we are seeking to find out what that person is trying to do in this life, including what he is trying to avoid, and what he is trying to be" (p. 112). The concept of personal strivings (Emmons, 1986, 1989, 1996), idiographically coherent patterns of goal strivings, was developed in order to describe what a person typically is trying to do. Personal strivings are rooted in Floyd Allport's (1937) concept of "teleonomic trends." Each individual can be characterized by a unique set of "trying to do" tendencies. For example, a person may be "Trying to appear attractive to the opposite sex," "Trying to be a good listener to friends," and "Trying to be better than others." Additional examples of strivings are presented in Table 2.1.

Note that these strivings are phrased in terms of what a person is "trying" to do, regardless of whether or not he or she is actually successful. For example, a person might be "Trying to get others to like me" without necessarily being successful. Strivings may be fairly broad, such as "Trying to make others happy," or more specific, such as "Trying to make my partner happy." Also, strivings may be either positive or negative. That is, they may be about something a person typically tries to obtain or keep, or about end-states that one typically tries to avoid or prevent. For example, a person might typically try to obtain respect from others, or might typically try to avoid others' disrespect. This difference in the framing of strivings along an approach–avoidance dimension appears to carry ramifications for goal-related affect, as discussed in the next chapter.

Referring to goals as "strivings" implies an action-oriented perspective on human motivation and stresses the behavioral movement toward identifiable end-points. After all, the term striving is a verb, implying vigorous exertion. Most definitions of goals similarly stress movement. For example, Kruglanski (1996) defines a goal as "a desirable state of affairs one intends to attain through action" (p. 600). However, one can also strive toward particular modes of being without necessarily making a strenuous effort, as in Eastern philosophies, which emphasize a cessation

TABLE 2.1. Examples of Personal Strivings
_____

"Find that special someone."
"Make sure everyone's needs are met."
"Avoid revealing too much of myself."
"Demonstrate my love to my children each day."
"Force men to be intimate in relationships."
"Treat my wife with respect and admiration."
"Avoid being dependent on my boyfriend."
"Win at all sports."
"Make it appear that I am intelligent."
"Avoid cleaning the kitchen."
"Become financially independent from others."
"Avoid destructive gossip."
"Overcome shyness around strangers."
"Make life easier for my parents."
"Do something spontaneously, once a week."
_____

Note. Strivings generated in response to the sentence stem: "I typically try to _____." Wording is original.

of striving and nonattachment to goals (e.g., "Being at peace with one-self," "Being at one with the universe"). Certainly, the notion of strivings (as a noun) would include these latter examples, in that they reflect desired end-points or objectives to be realized. Chapter 5 reveals that spiritual concerns are reflected in both "doing" and "being" goals; indeed, perhaps that is an important distinction between the types of goals that adherents to Western and Eastern religious systems aspire toward.

   Personal strivings can be thought of as superordinate abstracting qualities that render a cluster of goals functionally equivalent for an individual, in other words, that place them into broad equivalence classes. In this sense, a striving is similar to the definition of a motive disposition. However, the critical difference lies in the idiographic nature of the personal striving. Each person's strivings are uniquely his or hers; no two people share the exact configuration of strivings. A personal striving is a unifying construct, uniting what may be phenotypically different goals or actions around a common quality or theme. A given striving can be achieved in a variety of ways and satisfied via any one of a number of concrete goals. Strivings serve as motivational organizing principles that lend coherence and continuity to day-to-day goal pursuits and to temporally extended states of mind such as possible selves (Sheldon & Kasser, 1995). More than a decade's worth of research has shown that they are a valid representation of how people structure and experience their lives. Strivings (and, for that matter, any of the other personal goal units) are critical constructs for understanding the ups and downs of everyday life.

The concept of personal strivings was envisioned as filling an existing gap in the conceptual framework of personality psychology. Strivings can be viewed as idiographic instantiations of motive dispositions, possessing more discriminativeness than motives yet more stability and consistency than projects or concerns. For example, a person with a high need for achievement may have separate strivings of "Trying to do a good job," "Trying to get things accomplished," or "Trying to get attention from others" and may believe that achieving is the best way to attain those objectives. However, less than half of strivings can be mapped onto the three major motivational systems of achievement, affiliation–intimacy, and power, suggesting that strivings are more than just concretized and contextualized versions of a small number of global motives.

Theoretical Moorings

Given the ubiquitousness of goals within psychology, it should not be surprising that the personal strivings construct is compatible with a number of different theoretical frameworks. I have already noted the centrality of the goal construct in evolutionary conceptions of human nature. At least two other theoretical orientations can be used to understand personal strivings within a larger framework of psychological functioning: cognitive personality theory as represented in the control theory of self-regulation (Carver & Scheier, 1998; Powers, 1973) and existential personality theory (Yalom, 1980).

According to the most widely accepted forms of control theory, various levels of reference values that regulate action exist in a hierarchy ranging from the narrowest, most specific actions to the broadest, most abstract principles. Behavior is a discrepancy-reduction process, whereby individuals act to minimize the discrepancy between their present condition and a desired standard or goal. Personal strivings can be thought of as one of these reference values that are used to guide action. Control theory is primarily concerned with the process of goal striving and the relation between goal striving and affective organismic consequences. Goals are dynamic entities that have a natural hierarchicality in their organization. Control theory assumes that goals and behaviors at lower levels in the hierarchy are subsumed under broader level, superordinate goals (Carver & Scheier, 1998).

Human actions always involve choice, and authentic choices presuppose that a person might make alternative choices. Existentialist perspectives (e.g., Yalom, 1980) emphasize the role of meaning and choice as the individual actively constructs his or her life circumstances. An individual creates goals among possibilities and, in the optimal situation, arranges them so as to achieve maximum meaning and satisfaction in life and minimal conflict between them. At the core of the existentialist position is directionality and choice. Personal strivings, as personalized goals, represent choices that individuals make as they direct their lives toward particular outcomes and away from others. Personal strivings constitute an important source of meaning as people's lives are structured around what they are trying to accomplish. Psychologists are beginning to warm to the concept of personal meaning (Wong & Fry, 1998), and Klinger (1998) persuasively argues that the construct of "meaning" has no meaning outside of a person's goals and purposes. The relation between goals and personal meaning is explored in Chapter 7. Changes in goals, discussed in that chapter, are represented by losses, additions, and shifts in goal hierarchies, and can be viewed as alterations in life meanings for the person (Baumeister, 1991).

Existentialism also provides a starting point for considering the nature of ultimate concerns in people's lives. An existential stance dominated the theology and philosophy of Paul Tillich, one of the great contributors to 20th-century thought. For Tillich (1951),

> Man is ultimately concerned about his being and meaning. "To be or not to be" in this sense is a matter of ultimate, unconditional total and infinite concern. Man is infinitely concerned about the infinity to which he belongs, from which he is separated, and for which he is longing . . . man is ultimately concerned about that which determines his ultimate destiny beyond all preliminary necessities and accidents. (p. 14)

As I contend in Chapter 5, and, indeed, throughout this volume, it is this concern with ultimacy that shapes and gives direction to one's most profound goal strivings.

Distinguishing between the Personal Goal Units

It can be confusing for readers who are not familiar with the goal literature to be confronted with several similar-sounding constructs. Near the end of their review, Austin and Vancouver (1996) size up the situation in the following way: "A proliferation of interrelated goal dimensions makes an examination of the goal construct problematic. There are too many putative dimensions floating around with minimal interconnections established empirically" (p. 361). One might add that interconnections need also be established *conceptually*. Are there substantive differences between each of these popular goal constructs? Or is this just another example of a phenomenon that psychologists are so competent at—designating different names for what essentially is the same thing? Although these constructs do share some common theoretical and methodological ground, there are important conceptual differences between them.

Current concerns refer to hypothetical latent states that underlie goal striving. Personal projects refer not to hypothetical states but to a set of related acts over time—the observable behavior that presumably corresponds to a concern. They are not what the person has, but rather what the person does. Little (1996) aligns the personal goal units along an internal–external continuum. Personal strivings, according to Little, reflect the internal, self-defining aspects of the person, whereas life tasks tend to reflect external, socially constructed, culturally mandated problems. Personal projects occupy middle ground along this continuum, reflecting both culturally prescribed shared developmental concerns as well as idiosyncratic "magnificent obsessions and trivial pursuits" (B. R. Little, 1989, p. 15). Life tasks focus on nontrivial problems that the individual wishes to solve. These tasks are rooted in developmental stages and could be viewed as a subset of concerns or projects that are made salient by life transitions that need to be accomplished by a person in a particular age and social group. Thus, these represent age-graded normative tasks and goals that are more contextually embedded than are concerns or strivings. Read and Miller (1989) point out that life tasks capture the organization of goals and strategies around specific periods and contexts in people's lives, and are less suited for describing individual differences more generally. A personal striving, defined as a class of goals that is characteristic for a particular person, describes enduring and recurring personality characteristics. Unlike current concerns and life tasks, the personal striving approach was not developed as a reaction against the motive-disposition approach and in fact, is quite compatible with it (Emmons, 1989). Strivings are enduring goals, or enduring concerns that presumably transcend particular developmental transition periods. As would be predicted, the personal goal research reports that, on average, a larger number of strivings than life tasks tend to be generated by subjects.

While such distinctions between the units are possible in principle, in reality the boundaries between them are often obscured. Clearly, there is considerable overlap among these goal constructs. Part of the difficulty lies in the ambiguously defined category breadth and time frame of the respective constructs.

Breadth of the construct (narrow and concrete versus broad and abstract) is important in that it defines the range of outcomes that are acceptable as goal attainments. For example, "Trying to get to know others better" may be satisfied by a wider range of outcomes than "Getting Sue to go to the dance." The majority of the goal units are not explicit with reference to category width. Life tasks may vary in scope, from "Becoming a good person" to "Getting good grades" (Cantor & Langston, 1989). According to B. R. Little (1989), projects can be defined at a microbehavioral and a macro-intentional level (e.g., "Going to church on Sunday" vs. "Growing in my relationship with the God of the universe"). Projects, tasks, and concerns can all vary between these extremes. Strivings, on the other hand, possess greater category breadth, as they are postulated to occupy a higher level in the hierarchy of motivational control (Emmons, 1989).

The characteristic level at which individuals define their life goals appears to be an important individual difference variable, with implications for the self-regulation of action. In control theory language, some individuals typically self-regulate using more abstract reference levels than other individuals (this involves the distinction between high- and low-level goals; see also Vallacher and Wegner, 1985, for individual differences in preferred levels of action identification). This difference is likely to have important ramifications for one's subjective experience, such as monitoring progress toward goals. The more abstract the goal is, the more difficult it will be to monitor progress toward it, and the more inconsistent will be the feedback. For example, it is relatively clear when one has achieved good grades, but how can one ever be really certain that one is a good person? Frese and Semmer (1985) speculate that depression may result from vague standards of success. For instance, an amorphous standard of "doing well" is vague enough that a person can decide after the fact that his or her performance is not good enough. In the next chapter, research on the relation between level of goal abstraction and psychological well-being is reviewed.

Time frame (term) is another important aspect of these personal goal units. Goals may be short-term, medium-term, or long-term. Although more abstract goals are typically viewed as more temporally extended than concrete goals, time frame can be independent of category breadth. For example, one could have a narrow, long-term goal (keep all of my pencils sharpened for the rest of my life) as well as broad, short-term goals (become a wise person by the end of the day).

What is the time frame of the personal goal units? Tasks are specific to a life-transition stage. They are relevant while the person is negotiating passage through the stage. Current concerns may last anywhere from a few moments to a lifetime, but have a clear onset and termination point. Personal projects may also range from short-term to long-term, but are also marked by clear beginning and end. Personal strivings, on the other hand, are assumed to be relatively enduring, although undoubtedly there is revision, abandonment, and redefinition of the striving throughout the life span. To my knowledge, there is no long-term longitudinal study of personal goals from which definitive statements on the degree of stability versus change in personal goal systems could be derived.

Assessing Personal Goals

The assessment of personal goals begins with having respondents freely generate a list of their concerns, tasks, projects, or strivings. In this initial step, the definition of the construct is given, usually with examples, and participants write down as many goals as they can within a specified time period, ranging from 10 minutes (projects) to an hour (strivings). Klinger's (1987) Interview Questionnaire (IntQ) requires participants to list their current concerns in 14 major life areas (friends, employment, family). Some of the categories are further subdivided and are accompanied by illustrative concerns. In personal projects analysis, participants are told that personal projects are activities and concerns that people have and are provided with examples such as "Completing my English essay" and "Getting more outdoor exercise" (B. R. Little, 1989). They are instructed to list all of the personal projects that they are engaged in or are thinking about at the time, and are told that these projects should represent everyday activities and concerns and not necessarily major life projects.

In the case of personal strivings, individuals are given the definition of a personal striving as "the things that you typically or characteristically are trying to do in your everyday behavior." They are then provided with several examples, such as "Trying to persuade others one is right" and "Trying to help others in need of help." It is stressed that these strivings are phrased in terms of what the person is "trying" to do, regardless of whether the person is actually successful. They are also instructed that the strivings may be either positive or negative, and that the striving must refer to a repeated, recurring goal, not to a one-time concern. Following generation of the strivings list, participants are asked to make a number of evaluative appraisals of each of their strivings on a series of rating scales, and are asked to complete a goal instrumentality matrix. The complete instructions for the elicitation and assessment of personal strivings are provided in Appendix A.

Do the instructions that are given to participants affect the nature of the goal units that are generated in the elicitation procedure? In an interesting recent study, Ware and Mendelsohn (1997) varied the instructions and examples used to elicit personal goals from respondents. They found that different numbers of goals were generated depending on the instructional set, and that variations in instructions and examples can affect the correlations between appraisal dimensions and criterion variables. In their study, striving instructions were compared with project instructions and a set of "minimalist" instructions that were labeled simply "goals." Striving instructions generated the largest number of units, and strivings were shown to predict self-esteem more strongly than did projects or general goals. This higher validity coefficient for strivings provides some indirect support for Little's (1996) thesis that strivings reflect more internal, self-defining aspects of personality. The Ware and Mendelsohn study holds significant implications for research on goals and well-being. Their study suggests that not all instructions mean the same thing, and that the assessment protocol makes a difference in the types of units obtained, how these units are appraised, and their relation to criterion variables such as well-being.

Personal Goal Dimensions: Striving Assessment Scales

Following elicitation of the personal goals, respondents are asked to rate each goal on several dimensions. The dimensions used in any one study depend on of the specific purposes of the research. Theoretically derived dimensions from the motivational literature include value, expectancy for success, instrumentality, and commitment. Other dimensions are included because of their presumed relevance to the particular study. For instance, Ruehlman and Wolchik (1988) successfully assessed perceived interpersonal support and hindrance associated with specific projects. Personal goal assessments typically exploit the power of a mixed nomothetic–idiographic research strategy. The units are individually tailored to the respondent, yet the ratings scales used for appraising the goals yield quantitative comparisons between different persons independent of idiosyncratic goal content. Goal construals typically account for more variance in well-being scores than does goal content (Emmons, 1996). A review of the goal-appraisal dimensions used in personal goals research can be found in Emmons (1997). Seventeen striving assessment dimensions are shown in Appendix A.

Striving Instrumentality Matrix

A number of investigators have pointed to the possibility of assessing the degree of intergoal conflict within the person's goal system. This can be accomplished by constructing for each person a matrix in which both the rows and columns list the person's goals. Respondents are asked to rate the degree of conflict–instrumentality between each pair of goals, until the entire matrix is filled out. Each goal is in effect rated twice, in terms of the effect that it has on other goals and the effect that other goals have on it. For the matrix as a whole, the average amount of conflict (or the inverse, instrumentality) in the person's goal system is determined and is used as a variable in between-subject analyses. Cox and Klinger (1988) have demonstrated the applicability of the instrumentality matrix for motivational counseling with alcoholics. Emmons and

King (1988) found that conflict measured in this fashion prospectively predicted high levels of negative affect, psychosomatic complaints, and physician visits over a 1-year period. This research is described in more depth in Chapter 4. The Striving Instrumentality Matrix is included in Appendix A.

Psychometric Properties

The personal goal approaches differ in the degree to which they have been concerned with formal psychometric considerations such as reliability and validity. Klinger (1987) made a compelling case for why traditional reliability estimates are only partially appropriate for both the content and dimensions of personal goals. Commitment to goals, particularly goals less central to the person, is likely to fluctuate over time. A lack of stability (a psychological process) need not imply lack of reliability (a psychometric situation). Internal consistency estimates are not wholly appropriate either. Since there is no assumption of homogeneity of goal content, there is no reason to expect high internal consistencies. Although such reliability values have been computed for various goal dimensions and have been shown to be acceptably high (Brunstein, 1993; Emmons & King, 1989; Sheldon & Kasser, 1995), the meaning of these is debatable.

Although acknowledging these difficulties, researchers have made some progress in estimating reliabilities of the goal measures. Both the stability of the goals themselves as well as the goal dimensions have been examined. Emmons (1986) computed both 3- and 6-month stability coefficients for the 18 striving assessment dimensions. The stabilities of the individual scales ranged from .58 to .91 for the 1-month interval (with a mean of .73), and from .47 to .70 for the 3-month period (with a mean of .60). Social desirability and importance were the most stable, while effort and impact were the least stable. Wadsworth and Ford (1983) reported 3-month stabilities of 12 goal dimensions ranging from .48 to .82, with a mean of .58. Cox and Klinger (1988) administered the IntQ to 42 alcoholic inpatients upon intake and 1 month later. The test–retest correlations of eight concern dimensions ranged from .07 to .77 with a mean of .30. Brunstein (1993; Brunstein, Danglemayer, & Schultheiss, 1996) reported 10-week stability coefficients ranging from .73 to .85 for the dimensions of commitment to and attainability of personal goals.

The stability of the goals themselves has also been investigated. In a sample of 40 undergraduates tested after 1 year, 82% of personal strivings listed at Time 1 were still present, with minor wording changes (Emmons, 1989). After 18 months, 45% were still present, and a 3-year follow up yielded a stability of just over 50%. Thus, there is evidence that strivings reflect enduring concerns in people's lives. Many of the 50% of personal strivings that were no longer present were associated with a particular life context (college environment) that was no longer part of the person's life.

Klinger (1987) had subjects take the IntQ 1 month apart and had them identify the concerns that were present at both times. For concerns that appeared only once, subjects indicated the reason, from forgetting to mention the concern to having attained the goal or abandoned pursuit of it. Thus, it was possible to estimate reliability by examining instability due to error. Nineteen percent of the concerns had been forgotten, or had become too trivial to mention. The remaining 81% were either still active or omitted for legitimate reasons (consummated or disengaged from during the period). This innovative approach suggests that the IntQ reliably assesses subjects' concerns.

In addition to examining the stability of specific goals, personal goal stability can also be examined at the goal-aggregate level. From this perspective, specific goals may drop in or out of a person's hierarchy, yet their concern with broader principles may persist. For example, the nature of power strivings may be very different when the person is in college as opposed to the corporate world. Yet there may still be continuity in terms of an overall concern with power. Cox and Klinger (1988) computed test–retest correlations on the mean proportion of concerns listed under various categories (e.g., interpersonal, health, religion). These correlations ranged from –.03 (alcohol-related concerns) to .75, with a mean of .38. In the 3-year follow-up of personal strivings, I (Emmons, 1989) have found stability correlations ranging from .47 to .88 for striving categories. Thus, although around one half of the individual strivings changed, there was impressive evidence of continuity on a broader level.

Thematic Coding of Goal Content

Strivings, as personal goals, are just that—*personal*. In research on strivings, I have tried to take the personal seriously, and not reduce strivings to global categories. Nevertheless, for certain research purposes, one may wish to examine strivings at a more aggregate level of analysis. For this reason, I developed a coding system for categorizing the target of what the person is striving for. This system allows researchers to move from an idiographic to a nomothetic level of analysis. The coding categories have been expanded over the years, while the coding criteria within each category have been occasionally refined to improve the reliability and validity of the system. Twelve of the categories useful in coding the aims of human strivings, with representative examples, are shown in Table 2.2. The entire coding system is reproduced in Appendix B.

The categories include the major motive classes of achievement, affiliation, intimacy, and power (McClelland, 1985), along with a number of other higher-order themes. The striving coding system clusters together strivings based on their surface similarities rather than on the basis of latent motivational themes. Research that has examined associations between the striving content categories and psychological well-being outcomes is presented in subsequent chapters.

GOAL ACCESSIBILITY: UNCONSCIOUS MOTIVATION AND SELF-DECEPTION

A concern that arose when I first began research on personal strivings pertained to the thorny issue of unconscious motivation. Mindful of the limitations of assessing motivation through conscious self-report, I have taken this concern seriously and have tried to form reasoned responses to it. An assumption in the direct assessment of goals is that people will be able to openly reflect on and accurately report their goals in a veridical, nondefensive manner. Goals are defined to be at a level of abstraction such that they can be easily articulated by the individual, although strivings may not be in conscious awareness when the person is actually working on them. Strivings are postulated to function in much the same manner as schemas, scripts, and other superordinate guiding structures (strivings could be conceived of as "MOPs"—motivational organizing principles). In addition, individual differences exist in the level of abstraction that subjects appear to prefer when describing their strivings. Some persons describe their strivings in high-level, self-reflective language, whereas others tend to report mostly lower-level, concrete concerns. Within a given individual, strivings are arranged hierarchically, and any of these may be activated into awareness depending on internal or external eliciting conditions.

What actually occurs when a person is asked to generate a list of personal goals? Where do defensive processes enter in? The process of generating and rating a goal list is open to a multitude of potentially distorting influences, including unconscious (or nonconscious) motivational factors and self- and other-deception. There are key issues that need to be addressed. For instance, do people harbor unconscious goals that they conceal from themselves or others? Do people deliberately alter their strivings according to self-presentational concerns? These dual considerations of deceiving others and self have long been of concern in the field of personality assessment.

Unconscious or nonconscious factors can affect both goal formation and goal striving. Generally, researchers studying goals and goal

TABLE 2.2. Personal Striving Coding Categories

1. *Approach–avoidance*
Goals that involve preventing or avoiding a negative, undesirable state of affairs (avoidant goals; e.g., "Avoid letting anything upset me," "Not to feel inferior in social gatherings").

2. *Achievement*
Concern with success, accomplishment, competing with a standard of excellence (e.g., "Realize my potential as far as a career is concerned," "Work toward higher athletic capabilities").

3. *Affiliation*
Concern with approval and acceptance, and preventing loneliness (e.g., "Be friendly to others so they will like me," "Meet new people through my present friends," "Avoid being left out").

4. *Intimacy*
Goals that express a desire for close, reciprocal relationships (e.g., "Help my friends and let them know I care," "Accept others as they are," "Try to be a good listener").

5. *Power*
Goals that express a desire to influence and impact others (e.g., "Force men to be intimate," "Be the best when with a group of people," "Make people laugh").

6. *Personal growth and health*
Goals that pertain to improving or maintaining mental and physical health (e.g., "Develop a positive self-worth," "Not eat between meals, to lose weight," "Learn new skills and apply old ones").

7. *Self-presentation*
Concern with making a favorable impression on others (e.g., "Appear intelligent to others," "Avoid appearing outrageous," "Make myself physically attractive").

8. *Independence*
Goals that express a desire for autonomy and self-assertion (e.g., "Be myself and not do things to please others," "Not be a pushover with others," "Be an individual").

9. *Self-defeating*
Strivings that reflect a lack of growth and/or harm to the self (e.g., "Be perfect at everything," "Do things that annoy others," "Avoid the truth when faced with unpleasant facts").

10. *Emotionality*
Strivings that focus on feelings and emotional regulation (e.g., "Be more considerate of Teresa's feelings," "Be honest with myself about how I truly feel," "Suppress my feelings/emotions").

11. *Generativity*
Strivings that reflect a desire for symbolic immortality (e.g., "Make a lasting contribution to my agency's mission," "Feel useful to society," "Make my life mean something").

12. *Spirituality*
Strivings that are oriented toward a search for the sacred (e.g., "Deepen my relationship with God," "Learn to tune into a higher power throughout the day," "Appreciate God's creations").

processes identify more with cognitive theory than with psychody-
namics. Thus, they have not been unduly concerned with unconscious
goals and unconscious conflict. Unlike its historical ancestors, contemporary motivation research places less emphasis on unconscious motives. The emerging consensus can be summed up in the following: While
goals may not be ordinarily represented in consciousness, people can,
when asked, give more or less accurate accounts of what they are trying
to accomplish. Although most goal research has focused on consciously
articulated concerns, there is no requirement that people be aware either
of the content of the goal or underlying goal processes, or, in the case of
evolutionary theory, the ultimate function of the goal pursuit (Buss,
1995). It is important to recognize that a number of factors affect the
ability of people to access goal-relevant information, not all of them motivated, defensive processes. For example, breadth of the construct (concrete vs. abstract), its position in the hierarchy of action (high- vs. low-
level), and goal content as opposed to goal process (such as conflict) all
influence accessibility to consciousness. It may turn out that level of consciousness may be a dimension of goals, with some goals dynamically
more available to awareness than others, but with even those less accessible becoming accessible under certain conditions. It is also likely that
the successful pursuit of goals requires that the person focus attention on
strategies for goal attainment rather than on a continuous reflection on
the content of the goal. Thus, inordinate attention on the actual goal
may inhibit adaptive goal-relevant problem solving.

Goal Accessibility and Information Processing

Social cognition researchers use the term "automatic" to distinguish unconscious goals from deliberate, conscious goals. Bargh and Barndollar's
(1996) model of automatic goal activation suggests that situational cues
trigger the activation of chronic, latent goals outside of a person's awareness. These "auto-motives" then guide behavior without the person being
aware of the influence of the guiding goal on thought, perception, action,
and emotion. Thus, people often engage in goal-directed actions without
consciously choosing, intending, or "trying" to do so. This is not a defensive process, but merely reflects normal operations of the information-
processing system. Without the need for conscious decision making, goal-
directed behavior can proceed more smoothly and effortlessly. Experimental studies using unobtrusive priming techniques have demonstrated
that the activation of social goals (affiliation) can affect subsequent
affiliative behavior (Bargh & Barndollar, 1996). Interestingly, though, the
effects of temporary goal priming were short lived; chronic goals and motives tended to exert more influence in later trials of the experiment.
    Although most strivings are likely to be proactive and chronic

rather than reactive and temporary, the auto-motive model would predict that certain strivings, particularly when frustrated, are likely to remain active for long periods of time outside of awareness. These strivings, then, might not appear on a list generated by the person in the striving assessment procedure, unless cued by mental representations of relevant environmental features. For instance, the striving "Make it appear that I am intelligent" might be triggered by a belief that the striving assessment, particularly when administered in a classroom setting, is in reality a measure of ability rather than personality. Such a belief might be activated by subtle cues conveyed by the researcher, who in this example may also be the instructor.

Perhaps the most comprehensive model of conscious and unconscious influences was proposed by Epstein (1994), who posited two parallel, interacting modes of information processing: the experiential and rational systems. The two systems operate according to different principles. The rational system is analytical, logical, and deliberative, and verbal, while the experiential system is intuitive, holistic, automatic, and nonverbal. Epstein argues that the experiential system should replace the Freudian concept of the unconscious, and marshals considerable evidence for its operation in diverse theories, laboratory research, and everyday life. Disputing the view of unconscious processes as irrational, Epstein argues for the adaptiveness of experiential processing in everyday decision making. Religion, interestingly, according to Epstein, provides some of the best evidence for the two modes of information processing. He argues that its cross-cultural universality stems from its ability to communicate with the experiential system. As religion speaks both to the heart and to the head, its appeal might lie in its ability to create harmony between the experiential and rational systems.

Personal striving, as all behavior, is the product of the joint operation of the two systems. Elsewhere (Emmons, 1989) I speculated that strivings satisfy three basic needs: safety and control, social belongingness, and self-esteem and competence. A person possesses implicit, preconsciously activated beliefs about how to best satisfy these needs (e.g., "In order to be loved, I must try to withhold my true feelings from others"). The core needs become transformed through experience into preconscious beliefs, which in turn lead to coherent patterns of goal striving. The transformation of implicit beliefs into conscious goals represents movement from the experiential to the rational mode of processing.

Self-Deception

The literature on self-deception may also offer some insights into nonconscious goal processes and nonconscious conflict. In their classic analysis of self-deception, Sackeim (1983) identified four criteria for self-deception: (1) Individuals hold two contradictory beliefs; (2) the beliefs are held simultaneously; (3) one of the beliefs is not subject to awareness; and (4) the self-deceptive process is motivated. Two general motives are believed to be served by self-deception: the avoidance of negative affect and the augmentation or protection of self-esteem (Sackeim, 1983).

Applying the concept to goal-directed behavior, self-deceptive processes could occur when individuals fail to recognize that they are committed to goals which might conflict with some other self-defining aspect. Sackeim (1983) states that self-deceptive processes are likely to be activated when individuals are confronted with an aspect of themselves that they find difficult to accept. Asking subjects to reflect on their innermost aspirations is clearly a self-confrontational condition that could activate self-deceptive processes. A person may refrain from thinking about and therefore reporting certain goals if they conflict with previously avowed goals. In addition, a pair of mutually exclusive goals might not be viewed as being in conflict because to recognize the conflict would force an inconsistency with a prior belief (that each goal is attainable). Either the person really believes each goal is attainable or deceives him- or herself into thinking that they are, which serves the purpose of avoiding negative affect associated with goal conflict. Defensive processes serve several purposes, one of which is to regulate painful affect associated with conflicting motivations. Thus, the assessment of conflicting goals may be problematic in that the existence of conflict itself may be ego-threatening. Nevertheless, the assessment of conscious conflict has proceeded and has yielded some important findings, which are presented in Chapter 4.

Implicit and Explicit Motivation: Two Systems?

Gordon Allport (1950) asserted that if one wanted to know what an individual was trying to do, all we need to do is to ask him or her. In stark contrast was Henry Murray (1938), who argued that motivation could be accessed only indirectly through fantasy. This debate over conscious and unconscious motivation has continued through the years and has given rise to a conception of motivational measures as drawing on two separate underlying systems: implicit motives and explicit motives. The term "implicit motives" applies to the types of needs Murray referred to. These needs are thought to be primitive, based on universal incentives and childhood experiences (e.g., McClelland, 1985). Implicit motives are biological and affective incentives that emerge early in life and operate outside of conscious awareness.

In contrast to implicit motives, explicit motives are largely conscious, cognitively elaborate, culturally determined (McClelland, Koestner, & Weinberger, 1989), and measured directly via self-report measures such as questionnaires. Importantly, questionnaire and projective measures of motivation tend to be unrelated to each other and to have different correlates. In other words, a person may score low on need for achievement in a fantasy-based measure such as the Thematic Apperception Test (TAT; Murray, 1938) but may report a high degree of achievement orientation when asked directly. In general, research has shown that questionnaire measures tend to predict self-conscious choices, particularly when the motive-relevance of a task has been made clear. On the other hand, projective measures tend to predict spontaneous behaviors that a person performs without being reminded of the motive-relevance of the task (McClelland et al., 1989). Evidently, self-report measures and thematic measures tap different underlying systems, one cognitive and conscious and the other motivational and unconscious.

As described earlier in this chapter, personal strivings can be coded with respect to the type of underlying motive disposition they seem to tap. The rationale behind this procedure involves the hierarchical ordering of implicit motives and explicit goals. Motives can be seen as clusters of recurrent prototypical goals in a fashion analogous to conceptualizing traits as clusters of prototypical behaviors (Emmons & McAdams, 1991), with personal strivings occupying the lower level of the hierarchy. Thus, personal goals occupy a place below social motives on a hierarchy of control (Powers, 1973). This hierarchy can be construed in a number of ways. The higher levels may be seen as less cognitive, less accessible to awareness and hence less self-conscious, less malleable, and less informed by situational particularities. On the other hand, at the next level, personal strivings may be seen as infused with the influences of motive dispositions, of beliefs and values, and of situational opportunity. Thus, personal strivings may be viewed as at once cognitive and motivational, as "secondary process" reflections of abstract, more basic needs. Although they exist at Level II in McAdams's (1995) three-tiered system, it is likely that they will empirically relate to constructs at Level I in much the same manner that characteristic adaptations might relate to basic tendencies in McCrae and Costa's (1996) model of personality.

Given the pervasive impact of motives on spontaneous thought and behavior, it seems reasonable to expect motives to find expression in individualized, self-generated goals. Emmons and McAdams (1991) found that personal goals, coded for motive content, did relate to the corresponding underlying motive. Following the standard striving protocol in that study, participants generated 15 strivings in response to the stem "I typically try to _____." These strivings were coded for relevance to achievement, affiliation, and power, using a scoring scheme adapted from the scoring procedures used for TAT stories. An individual who was high in need for power might have the daily goals to "Persuade others to my point of view" or to "Always get my way." In a similar type of study, King (1995) found that autobiographical memories, wishes, daily goals, and TAT-scored motives were largely unrelated to each other. In that study, the method used to measure a motive was the strongest link between the various motive measures.

In an important recent pair of studies, Brunstein, Schultheiss, and Graessman (1998) examined the relation between motives and goals in the prediction of well-being. They distinguished between motive-congruent goals and motive-incongruent goals within the domains of agency and communion. Progress toward motive-congruent goals predicted positive mood more strongly than did progress toward motive-incongruent goals. In support of the dual-system theory of motivation, the authors interpret their findings to suggest that the implicit motivational system monitors progress toward consciously articulated explicit goals. Their investigations indicated that motive dispositions combine with personal goals to influence affective well-being. In the next chapter, the literature on goals and well-being is comprehensively reviewed.

CONCLUSIONS

Some years ago, the social psychologist Bernard Weiner (1986) stated that the royal road to the unconscious may be less valuable than the dirt road to consciousness. I have found much inspiration in this saying. By asking participants directly about their goals and taking their descriptions at face value, considerable progress has been made in understanding the role of personal goal strivings in long-term levels of subjective well-being. This research forms the centerpiece of the next chapter.

CHAPTER THREE

Personal Goals and Subjective Well-Being

*A*ttempts to provide scientifically based answers to the question of who is happy and why typically invoke some conception of personality, motivation, or both. In their review of the characteristics of happy people, Myers and Diener (1995) argue that personality is a prime determinant of long-term happiness and well-being. A recent meta-analysis (DeNeve & Cooper, 1998) suggested that goal strivings represent additional personality influences on well-being. Myers and Diener (1995) conclude that there are three principles that theories of happiness must take into account: (1) Due to adaptation, the influence of life events is short-lived; (2) these life events must be interpreted within a cultural worldview that renders them as sources of suffering or as opportunities for growth; and (3) people's values and goals are potent contributors to their overall levels of happiness. It is the third point that Myers and Diener make that has been the focus of much of my research on personal strivings. This chapter is concerned with the role of personal motivation as an influence on long-term levels of happiness, or what has come to be known in the research literature as *subjective well-being*.

A substantial research base has been building for several years that, taken as a whole, demonstrates that people's priorities, goals, and concerns adequately account for variation in people's overall subjective well-being. Beyond this generalization, however, more specific questions can be posed. Are there certain types of goals that consistently are linked with happiness? To negative affect? To life satisfaction or meaning in life? Do the ways in which people strive for their goals, for example, by framing the goal in abstract or concrete terms, or by using approach versus avoidance language, affect the experience of well-being? Do the goals need to be integrated into a more or less coherent package for

43

maximal positive emotional consequences? What advice could be given
to persons so that they might more effectively regulate their behavior
around their goals? Can goals provide a sense of purpose and life meaning even in the absence of hedonic happiness? These are questions that
goal research into emotional well-being has begun to address in the past
decade. The purpose of this chapter is to summarize and synthesize the
existing literature, and suggest ways in which a goal framework may
have utility for addressing issues of fundamental human significance.

THE COMPONENTS OF SUBJECTIVE WELL-BEING

Subjective well-being refers to general long-term affective states of emotional well-being as well as cognitive states of life satisfaction and meaning in life. Research on the structure of well-being has reliably identified
three components: positive affect or pleasant emotions, negative affect
or unpleasant emotions, and a cognitive component of life satisfaction.
Positive affect reflects a person's level of pleasurable engagement with
the world, and negative affect is an indicator of a person's level of subjective distress (Watson & Tellegen, 1985). One of the major findings to
emerge from the subjective well-being literature in the 1980s was the discovery that long-term positive and negative affective states were relatively independent of each other in peoples lives. Much debate has
centered around the relationship between positive and negative affect
(Zautra, Potter, & Reich, 1998). The upshot of this is that positive and
negative emotions need to be measured separately in research on well-
being. It cannot be assumed that the presence of one indicates the absence of the other. Mental health problems are often defined by the negative pole of psychological functioning, in terms of stress, anxiety,
depression, alienation, and the like. However, a person may show little
sign of psychic distress yet still be dissatisfied and functioning sub-
optimally if he or she is living a life bereft of pleasant emotional experiences. Life satisfaction, the cognitive aspect of well-being, is a "global
evaluation by the person of his or her life" (Lucas, Diener, & Suh, 1996,
p. 616), indicating how close a person's actual life is to his or her conception of the ideal. Life satisfaction is only moderately correlated with
the positive and negative affective components of well-being, with absolute values ranging between .20 and .40. Research on goals and well-
being has recognized this multidimensional nature of well-being and typically attempts to measure its multiple components, though not all aspects have been measured in every study. Different components of well-
being tend to be associated with different aspects of goal systems.

Personal Goals and Subjective Well-Being

Within the domain of well-being, characteristics of personal goal systems have been explored as precursors of life satisfaction and long-term positive and negative affective states (Brunstein, 1993; Diener & Fujita, 1995; Emmons, 1986; B. R. Little, 1989; Omodei & Wearing, 1990; Yetim, 1993). Research on personal goals has shown that the possession of and progression toward important life goals are intimately tied to long-term well-being. Affect reflects the status of our goal pursuits. Our lives are structured around the pursuit of incentives that reflect fundamental human needs. Ryan (1995) contends that goals instantiate the needs for autonomy, competence, and relatedness and that an individual's sense of well-being depends upon the ability of the individual to make progress toward goals that fulfill these fundamental human needs.

One of the clearest examples of affective influences on goals comes from research on self-defining memories (Singer & Salovey, 1993). Within a master framework for memory, emotion, and personality, self-defining memories are a pivotal unit of analysis. These memories are a subset of autobiographical memories that are affectively intense, vividly recalled, and repetitively experienced. What determines affective intensity? The affective intensity and quality of a personal memory is determined, in part, by the relevance of that memory to the person's ongoing goal concerns. The greater the link between the memory and a current or future goal, the stronger the affect experienced when a memory is retrieved. Personal memories serve an integrating function; they serve to connect the past with the present and future, thus providing narrative coherence. Memories are also motivating: memories of successful goal attainment or, conversely, of failed efforts to secure a desired outcome can influence what people decide really matters in life and is worth investing in.

Over the past dozen years, the heuristic value of personal strivings in predicting levels of affective, cognitive, and physical well-being (Emmons, 1986, 1992; Emmons & King, 1988; see Emmons, 1996, for a review) has been established. Emmons (1996) organized the research findings on personal goals and well-being into three primary domains: goal content (what a person is trying to do, as, for example, striving for achievement or intimacy-related outcomes), goal orientation (how the person typically frames goals, as, for example, in approach or avoidance terms), and goal parameters (e.g., structural properties of goal systems, as, for example, conflict or differentiation between goals). Before I present an overview of the main findings from each of these respective areas, a digression is required in order to first describe how subjective well-being is typically measured in goal research.

Measuring Subjective Well-Being

As described earlier, subjective well-being contains both cognitive (life satisfaction and meaning) and emotional or affective components (positive and negative affect). In research on personal strivings and well-being, we have utilized a variety of self-report measures and reports from knowledgeable informants to assess these dimensions of well-being. One of the most commonly used procedures that we have employed is the daily mood report, an adjective checklist that participants complete on a daily basis for varying periods of time ranging from 2 weeks to 2 months. The mood adjectives were taken from earlier factor-analytic work in which certain terms loaded highest on two orthogonal factors (Diener & Emmons, 1984). Negative affect is measured by summing the ratings of depressed, unhappy, frustrated, worried/anxious, and angry/hostile, and positive affect by summing the ratings on happy, joyful, enjoyment/fun, and pleased. Aggregating mood measures over this time period results in a highly stable estimate of long-term levels of affective well-being. These composite scales have temporal reliability and internal consistency coefficients that approach .90 (Diener & Emmons, 1984). By altering the time frame, trait-like estimates of well-being can be provided for any specified time period, typically for the previous month, or, in some cases, as long as the entire previous year.

To minimize potential self-report biases such as memory distortion, we have in the past also employed an experience sampling procedure, or "beeper" methodology. Each subject is outfitted with a device, either a wristwatch or a pager, preset to sound an alarm at random times during the subject's waking hours. This method eliminates recall biases that can introduce measurement noise in retrospective accounts of well-being.

The cognitive component of well-being, life satisfaction, is often measured with the Satisfaction With Life Scale (SWLS; Diener, Emmons, Larsen, & Griffin, 1985), a brief and highly reliable evaluation of one's life as a whole. Widely employed in both clinical and nonclinical samples, evidence for the reliability and validity of the SWLS is available in Pavot and Diener (1993). Other goal research (e.g., Kasser & Ryan, 1993, 1996) has employed various other trait indices of well-being, including measures of vitality, self-actualization, self-esteem, and openness to experience. Vitality, recently introduced by Ryan and Frederick (1997), is "the subjective feeling of aliveness and energy" (p. 530). Subjective vitality correlates moderately with both positive and negative affect. From a measurement point of view, the choice of what precise measure to employ is not terribly critical, since empirical research has shown that the majority of these indices tender to cluster together (Compton, Smith,

Cornish, & Qualls, 1996; however, see Ryff, 1989, and Ryff & Singer, 1998, for an alternative perspective).

In a number of studies we have also gathered information from knowledgeable informants, or what is sometimes referred to as peer or observer reports. The term peer report originated within the person perception literature in social psychology and is technically misleading when applied in the subjective well-being research literature. Typically the report is from a significant member of the target person's social network. Virtually anyone knowledgeable may be asked to provide an appraisal of the person's typical levels of emotional well-being or life satisfaction, which include not only peers but also progeny, parents, professors, and pastors. Diener (1995) describes the strengths and limitations of reports provided by informants. Once aggregated, they can provide reliable and valid information, particularly on the elements of well-being that are most visible to an observer.

GOAL CONTENT AND SUBJECTIVE WELL-BEING

One way to examine the relation between personal goals and well-being is in terms of goal content. Is the content of what people are trying to do related to their level of well-being? Or are all goals created equal? To examine this issue using personal strivings we must move from an idiographic to a nomothetic level of analysis. As I described in the previous chapter, this move is made possible when strivings are coded into broader, thematic categories, such as achievement, power, generativity, and intimacy and the other themes displayed in Table 2.2. What are the affective consequences of pursuing different types of goals? I have summarized the findings from several studies in Table 3.1.

In general, the associations between striving content and well-being

TABLE 3.1. Goal Predictors of Subjective Well-Being

Related to positive indicators of well-being	Related to negative indicators of well-being
Affiliation–intimacy goals	Power goals
Spiritual goals	Extrinsic goals
Generativity goals	Goal conflict
Intrinsic goals	Goal ambivalence
Approach goals	Avoidant goals
Lower-level goals	Higher-level goals
Goal commitment	Interpersonal goal hindrance
Goal progress	

indicators have been modest, with most correlations ranging in the low to mid-.20s. In a number of different samples, we have found that the proportion of intimacy strivings in a person's striving system predicts greater levels of positive well-being, while the proportion of power strivings tends to be related to lower levels of positive well-being (see Emmons, 1996, for a review of the literature on striving type and well-being). Intimacy strivings reflect a concern for establishing deep and mutually gratifying relationships, whereas power strivings reflect a desire to influence others and have an impact on them. Generativity strivings, defined as those strivings that involve creating, giving of oneself to others, and having an influence on future generations (McAdams & de St. Aubin, 1992) also relate to higher levels of life satisfaction and to measures of positive affectivity. This suggests that if power motivation can be channeled into generative concerns, its potential harmful effects on well-being can be mitigated. That intimacy strivings should be related to higher levels of well-being should come as no surprise. The ability to engage in close intimate relationships is the hallmark of psychosocial maturity and a key component to psychological growth, according to a variety of theorists. Persons who are primarily power-oriented and possess many agentic strivings—to impress and/or control others—may experience less positive well-being for the converse reason, namely, that they are overinvested in individual striving to the exclusion of developing interdependent strivings. People with a predominance of power strivings in their goal hierarchies may also be committing their lives primarily to obtaining extrinsic sources of satisfaction, to which we turn next.

Power-oriented individuals are likely to possess materialistic strivings, and materialism has been repeatedly shown to detract from well-being (Ahuvia & Friedman, 1998). Kasser and Ryan (1993, 1996) demonstrated that the rated importance of extrinsically oriented goals of achieving financial success, social recognition, and physical attractiveness were negatively related to several measures of well-being, including vitality and self-actualization. Additionally, in the latter study the rated importance of these goals was positively associated with measures of anxiety, depression, narcissism, and physical symptomatology. Alternatively, subjects who possessed the intrinsic goals of personal growth and community contribution reported higher levels of well-being. The authors concluded that there is a "dark side to the American dream"—that a relative emphasis on fame, fortune, and success to the neglect of intrinsically meaningful goals is more likely to lead to psychological and interpersonal problems. This appears to be true, even when the current perceived attainment of these goals is high (Sheldon & Kasser, 1998). Sheldon and Kasser showed in a 12-week longitudinal study that goal attainment toward intrinsic goals enhanced well-being, whereas progress toward extrinsic goals was unrelated to well-being. When it comes to psychological well-being, what people are striving for—the content of their aims and ambitions—does matter. Not all goals *are* created equal, and not all goal attainment is equally healthy. At first glance, this might seem blatantly obvious, yet goal theories of affect have been known to indiscriminately equate goal attainment with positive affective outcomes, regardless of goal content (Locke & Kristof, 1996).

Materialistic goal influences on well-being were also examined by Diener and Fujita (1995), who proposed that personal strivings mediate the relation between resources and well-being. Beginning with different assumptions than Kasser and Ryan, they hypothesized that resources such as money, good looks, health, or intelligence should be related to well-being *only* to the extent to which these resources enable the individual's personal strivings. Subjects rated the relevance of each of 21 resources for the attainment of each of their strivings. The degree to which various resources were possessed by the subjects was based on judgments by knowledgeable informants rather than through self-reports. Significant correlations were found between goal relevance of resources and negative affect and life satisfaction; higher correlations were also observed between goal-relevant resources and well-being than between less relevant resources and well-being. The possession of resources per se, independent of goal strivings, was unrelated to well-being. Thus, the greater the congruence between a person's goals and his or her resources, the higher the well-being that person tends to experience. It is interesting to note that consistent with the research of Kasser and Ryan cited earlier, the "intrinsic" resources of self-confidence, social skills, and self-discipline received the highest relevance ratings, whereas the "extrinsic" resources of material possessions, physical attractiveness, and money were rated as mostly irrelevant to the attainment of one's goals. Both studies seriously question that the "American dream" of fame, fortune, and image is a desirable state of affairs to strive toward; in reality, it may present not a dream but a nightmare. Yet the latter class of goals remain a powerful draw in the lives of many people, despite its inability to provide lasting satisfaction. This situation suggests that either people's implicit theories of the types of outcomes that will lead to happiness is wrong, or that anticipated happiness and satisfaction are not the primary motivations for establishing and pursuing goals. Happiness may often be pursued in the marketplace in a consumer culture, yet that appears to be the wrong place.

Despite these important studies, relatively little research in the personal goal literature has examined the relationship between the content of personal goals and well-being indicators. Rarely have studies on goal content and well-being included non-college based samples. One exception is the work of Rapkin and Fischer (1992). In an elderly community sample, these authors found that elders leading satisfied lives were most concerned with the maintenance of social goals, whereas disengagement from social roles and relationships was associated with higher levels of depression. In another study involving elderly respondents (mean age = 75), Lapierre, Bouffard, and Bastin (1997) found that social contact goals were linked with greater satisfaction and meaning in life, whereas health preservation goals were associated with dissatisfaction and a lack of meaning. This cross-sectional study was unable to determine the direction of causal influence, however.

Life Event Interactional Models

In addition to examining the main effect of goal type on well-being, a few studies have tested interactional models in which well-being is predicted to be dependent on the interaction between goals and stressful life events that impinge upon these goals. Much of this work has been implicitly or explicitly rooted in a transactional framework of stress and coping (Lazarus, 1993). In such an approach, chronic goal concerns are seen as mediators determining the relevance of objective life events for subjective well-being. Emmons (1991) proposed that life events are appraised with respect to the significance they hold for an individual's personal strivings, and that people attach significance to events that have implications for their strivings. This general hypothesis was supported in a study of daily life events and mood (Emmons, 1991). The degree to which individuals experienced positive and negative moods on a day-to-day basis was contingent upon positive and negative life events in domains relevant to their goals. Subjects completed daily goal lists and also took part in a daily mood study in which they completed mood forms twice every day for 21 days. On each form they noted the most important events of the day and rated their current mood. Personal strivings were coded for relevance to achievement, power, and affiliation. The events that were listed each day were categorized for their achievement or interpersonal content. For example, the moods of affiliative and intimacy-oriented individuals were most affected by interpersonal events, and achievement-oriented individuals were most susceptible to academic and task-related events. Results showed that having a large number of power-related daily goals was related to poorer subjective well-being. In addition, individuals whose goals were more achievement related tended to respond more strongly to achievement events. Thus, there was a correspondence between goal themes and the type of event to which subjects were most responsive. Similarly, Lavallee and Campbell (1995) found that self-relevant negative events (which they defined as those that adversely impinged upon personal goals) are more threatening to the self-concept and led to more self-focused attention and rumination. Thus, in addition to what a person is trying to do, the degree to which the environment facilitates or impedes goal striving cannot be ignored as a potent influence on well-being.

GOAL ORIENTATION AND WELL-BEING

A second way to examine how personal goals relate to well-being is through goal orientation. Goal orientation refers to individual differences in the manner in which goals are represented consciously by the individual and described linguistically when communicating these goals to others. Thus, orientation refers to individual differences in the mental representations of goals. Although it might be argued that this distinction is purely a semantic one, with no practical significance, it does appear that there are psychological benefits (and conversely, psychological costs) associated with different forms of goal framing. Goal orientations have been identified with respect to both goal setting and goal striving. Ford (1992) described several dimensions along which people vary in their general orientation to goals. The first dimension, active–reactive, describes differences in the degree to which goals are self-chosen by the individual versus imposed by external circumstances. In this sense, it shares conceptual ground with Deci and Ryan's (1985) intrinsic versus extrinsic orientation. Approach–avoidance refers to whether goals are conceptualized as positive incentives to be sought after or negative consequences to be avoided. Research linking variations in this orientation with well-being is described later in this chapter. A third dimension described by Ford is that of maintenance versus change: Does the person generally strive for change and growth in his or her goal system or is the person more concerned with maintaining the status quo? I have not attempted to assess this orientation in personal strivings.

We have been concerned primarily with measuring the effects of two orientations: level of goal abstraction and approach versus avoidance striving. A cursory review of research relevant to these two orientations follows. The interested reader is encouraged to consult the original publications for additional details.

Level of Abstraction

Waterman (1993) has identified two pathways by which individuals develop a sense of identity. Some people are satisfied with merely finding something to do, while others strive to find someone to be. When applied to personal goals, this orientation describes differences in level of goal specification. In examining strivings that subjects have spontaneously generated in past studies, it became apparent that people frame their goals at various levels of generality. Some individuals describe their goals in primarily broad, abstract, and expansive ways. They are concerned with being someone. Others tend to frame their goals in concrete, specific, and more superficial terms. They are concerned with finding something to do. Whereas one person's goal may be striving to "Learn about God's word," another's may be trying to simply "Memorize a verse of Scripture daily." Although these are ostensibly similar goals, they are framed at different levels of abstraction. "Keep my books straightened on my shelves" and "Write 10 pages a day for my new book" are low-level goals, whereas "Be an organized person" and "Try to make a contribution to future generations" are examples of higher level strivings. Table 3.2 shows goals characteristic of high- and low-level strivers.

This distinction between high- and low-level goals is reminiscent of the levels of Vallacher and Wegner's (1985) action identification theory, in which actions can be identified at various levels of analysis, ranging from the molecular to the molar (see Emmons, 1989, for a detailed comparison of personal strivings approach and action identification theory). There is considerable support for the notion of levels of abstraction within many different areas of psychology, including personality, clinical, social, and cognitive psychology. Cutting across these areas, levels of abstraction can be viewed within control theory (Carver & Scheier, 1998; Hyland, 1988; Powers, 1973). Control theory formulations posit a hierarchy of levels of control, with various levels of standards or goals arranged from the most concrete and narrow to the broadest and most abstract organizing principles. The lowest levels indicate how the action is to be carried out, while the higher levels provide information on the purposes or implications of the action. Goals or standards can be characterized at different levels within this hierarchy. People may be said to differ in terms of the level at which they tend to characterize their goals within the hierarchy. However, within the control theory literature, interest is lacking in individual differences in tendencies to phrase goals at different levels of abstraction.

In a study on striving level and well-being (Emmons, 1992), subjects in three samples generated lists of their personal strivings, which were then coded for level of abstraction according to the guidelines in the Personal Striving Coding Manual (see Appendix B). High-level strivings were described as being abstract, reflective, self-scrutinizing, and mentioning of internal states (moods, motives, thoughts). Low-level strivings were de-

TABLE 3.2. High- and Low-Level Strivers

High-level striver

"Treat others with dignity."
"Deepen my relationship to God."
"Be totally honest."
"Express my feelings to close friends and family openly and honestly."
"Be humble."
"Discern and follow God's will for my life."
"Expose my faith to others without offending them or pushing it on them."
"Keep positive thoughts in my mind."
"Make others feel good about themselves."
"Express to people that I love them."
"Compete against myself rather than others."
"Increase my knowledge of the world."

Low-level striver

"Look well–groomed and clean cut."
"Be funny and make others laugh."
"Speak clearly and straightforwardly to strangers."
"Look physically conditioned and physically fit."
"Keep good posture/walk straight."
"Look attentive and not bored in class."
"Use proper language and manners around adults and attractive girls."
"Make myself noticeable."
"Work hard (or at least make it look like it)."
"Be organized and neat, always have a clean room and a made bed."

Note. Adapted from Emmons (1992). Copyright 1992 by the American Psychological Association. Adapted by permission.

scribed as being more behavioral, more concrete and specific, and less self-reflective. All subjects completed a variety of psychological and physical well-being measures. Some of these were multiple measures over time using experience sampling and daily report methodology, whereas others were single-session questionnaire measures. Results revealed that high-level striving tended to be associated with psychological distress, particularly anxiety and depression. Low-level striving, on the other hand, was associated with greater levels of psychological well-being but also with more physical illness. I have referred to this pattern as the "illness versus depression" tradeoff. Among one subject's strivings in the study were the following: "Cut down on frozen dinners," "Have breakfast everyday," "Drink more water," "Improve my diet," "Shop for untainted fruits and vegetables," and "Cook without salt." Obviously all converging on a common theme, this subject turned out to report the lowest negative affect in the sample (0.5 on a 6-point scale); her positive affect score was well above the mean. Despite the best of intentions, she also scored above average on a measure of illness behavior, physician visits. In contrast, compare the strivings from this person: "Appear knowledgeable on any and all subjects to others," "Give others what I think they want from me," "Be the great mediator," "Look at matters realistically," and "Be understanding of others." This high-level striver scored two standard deviations above the mean on negative affect. What is reflected in the difference between these two is a tradeoff described by B. R. Little (1989) between having manageable versus meaningful goals, or more colorfully as "magnificent obsessions versus trivial pursuits" (B. R. Little, 1989). The most adaptive form of self-regulatory behavior may be to select concrete, manageable goals that are linked to personally meaningful, higher-order representations. High-level goals are rated as more important and more self-defining than are low-level goals. They carry vital information about what a person finds valuable, meaningful, and purposeful.

High-level goals are meaningful but also may be very difficult to accomplish. Because of their inherent fuzziness, it may be difficult to engage in progress monitoring. By fuzziness, I mean that clear markers of successful outcomes may be absent. To take one example from Table 3.1, how would one estimate success at "Deepening my relationship to God"? Without a clear idea of what needs to be done and without a yardstick to gauge progress by, the link between goal attainment and positive affective outcomes becomes more tenuous. In general, high-level goals are in fact rated as more difficult to accomplish and lower in clarity of means to accomplish them, thus potentially accounting for their link to negative affectivity. The logic of control theory would also predict a link between high-level goals and negative affect. Higher-order feedback systems have longer time lags for discrepancies to be reduced (Carver & Scheier, 1998). Negative affect is presumed to result from slower than desired progress toward one's goals. Thus, a longer time lag would increase the likelihood that the individual would experience emotionally distressing states. Conversely, we may be buffered from feeling bad if we fail to make progress toward high-level goals.

Low-level, concrete goals, particularly those devoid of emotional self-awareness, may be linked to physical illness through mechanisms of repressive-defensiveness. Repressiveness as a personality trait is characterized by the avoidance of emotionally threatening information. Low-level striving may be a way of distracting oneself. Presented with the psychologically charged task of confronting one's innermost aspirations, repressors are likely to find the task threatening, engage in avoidant processing, and produce less revealing and more superficial goals. If low-level striving is indicative of a repressive personality, then low-level strivers should also appraise their strivings more positively then high-level strivers, as repressors are prone to denying negative characteristics in themselves.

In order to test this hypothesis, Gomersall (1993) explored the relation between personal striving system variables (including level) and repressive-defensiveness. Repressors, as measured by the combination of scores on defensiveness and anxiety, had fewer strivings with emotional content and fewer negative, avoidant strivings (described in the next section) than did nonrepressors. Repressors also rated themselves as being more satisfied with the degree of progress made toward their strivings, rated their strivings as less difficult, and reported higher levels of instrumentality among their strivings. Examples of strivings reported by repressors include "Think positive about myself," "Not be quick to anger because it is not a good feeling," "Not show negative emotions so much," "Please people," and "Seek other people's approval." The theme of emotional avoidance is prevalent throughout these strivings, as is the need for social approval. The fact that repressors have insight into their mood regulation strategies suggests that avoidance is not an entirely unconscious process. It is also interesting that it is the emotionality component of the levels construct that is responsible for the links with repressive coping. There is a substantial literature on avoidant coping styles, autonomic arousal, and physical health (Weinberger, 1990, provided a scholarly review of repression as a personality trait) which implicates repressiveness as a risk factor for various physical illnesses.

A recent study provides additional evidence that striving level may be tapping differences in coping with threat and uncertainty. In this study (Orias, Leung, Dosanj, & Sheposh, 1998) high- and low-level strivers responded to a self-reflection task in which they selected questions about traits that varied in degree of diagnosticity. High-level strivers were found to seek out more diagnostic information about themselves than were low-level strivers, providing further support that high-level strivers are more reflective than are their more concrete counterparts.

Approach and Avoidant Goals

A second goal orientation that has been the focus of increasing research efforts in the personal goal literature is the degree to which individuals are striving for positive, approach goals rather than striving to avoid negative, aversive goals (Cochran & Tesser, 1996; Elliot & Sheldon, 1997; Elliot & Sheldon, 1998; Elliot, Sheldon, & Church, 1997; Emmons & Kaiser, 1996). The primary difference has to do with the regulatory focus of the goal. Approach goals are positive incentives to be sought after and moved toward, while avoidant goals are negative consequences to be avoided or prevented. The difference between approach and avoidant goals has to do with whether positive or negative outcomes are used as a benchmark for self-regulatory activity: for instance, trying to "Spend time with others" versus trying to "Avoid being lonely," or trying to "Avoid letting anything upset me" versus trying to "Stay calm even under difficult circumstances." The motivation literature (e.g., fear of failure vs. motive to approach success) has demonstrated that these differing orientations lead to very different behavioral patterns and consequences, even when similar goal content is involved (Elliot & Sheldon, 1998; Klinger, 1977). The majority of evidence suggests that avoidant striving is a less effective form of self-regulation relative to approach striving.

Emmons and Kaiser (1996) investigated the relation between approach and avoidance strivings and indicators of psychological and physical well-being. They predicted that individuals whose striving lists contain a large number of avoidant strivings will experience more psychological distress, particularly anxiety, than individuals whose lists predominantly include approach strivings. After completing the Personal Striving Assessment Packet (Emmons, 1989) subjects completed either a daily mood report for periods ranging from 3 to 6 weeks or a global measure of positive and negative affect. Subjects completed physical symptom reports in a similar manner, by indicating whether or not they had experienced any physical symptoms (eight categories) on the daily form. Subjects in all samples completed a number of well-being questionnaires.

The open-ended lists of strivings were coded for approach–avoidance according to the guidelines in the Personal Striving Coding Manual. Examples of avoidant strivings are shown in Table 3.3. As predicted, individuals with a large number of avoidant strivings experienced more psychological distress, particularly anxiety, than individuals with predominantly appetitive striving systems. Negative or inhibitory strivings appear to be a risk factor for psychological and physical distress, although in some cases they may lead to more effective self-regulation (Cochran & Tesser, 1996). Other data that we have collected suggests that avoidant strivings may play a role in interpersonal as well as intrapersonal satisfaction. In a sample of married couples (King & Emmons, 1991) we found that marital satisfaction was significantly negatively related to the proportion of the spouse's avoidant strivings. A person is likely to be less satisfied with his or her marriage if his or her spouse is predominantly concerned with avoiding negative outcomes. Thus, avoidant striving appears to exact an interpersonal as well as an intrapersonal toll on well-being. A more rigorous test of the link between avoidance personal goals and physical health was conducted by Elliot and Sheldon (1998). They found that avoidant personal goals are associated with increased physical

TABLE 3.3. Examples of Avoidant Goal Strivers

Person A

"Curb my habit of telling my personal thoughts and opinions to people I
    just meet."
"Share everything with my family."
"Not get angry at myself for being out of shape."
"Not have so many expectations of my son."
"Be a friend to my friends."
"Avoid feeling guilt."
"Curb my desire to spend money."
"Avoid comparing myself to my sister."
"Avoid the overwhelming feeling of wondering if my father approves
    of my decisions."

Person B

"Avoid offending others by maintaining my distance."
"Avoid taking sides in an issue, even though I may feel very strongly about
    one side."
"Avoid eye contact with strangers."
"Avoid arguments and even spirited discussions."
"Avoid engaging in a searching, serious discussion of issues."

Note. Adapted from Emmons (1996). Copyright 1996 by The Guilford Press. Adapted by per
mission.

symptomatology, both retrospectively and longitudinally. Furthermore,
mediational analyses revealed that perceived competence and perceived
controlledness mediated the relationship between avoidant striving and
subsequent ill health.

A number of mechanisms may be responsible for the association between avoidant strivings and psychological distress. I will briefly consider three: cognitive, motivational, and biological explanations. I make
no presumptions that these three are exhaustive, competing, or mutually
exclusive, nor do sufficient data currently exist to choose among them.
Some combination of these three, or other unidentified mechanisms,
may be ultimately required to fully delineate the relation between
avoidant strivings and suboptimal functioning.

Cognitively, trying to approach a desired outcome and trying to
avoid an undesired one appear to involve different information-
processing mechanisms. Schwarz (1990) proposed that it is the asymme-
try of approach and avoidance situations which leads to their different
emotional outcomes. According to Schwarz, in order to obtain a certain
positive outcome, there need be only a single accessible route to that
goal. However, in order to avoid or prevent an undesired outcome from
happening, all possible routes to that goals must be identified and

blocked. For instance the striving to "Avoid offending others by maintaining my distance" requires the individual to be constantly monitoring ongoing interactions for signs of negative reactions from others and making adjustments as needed. On the other hand, if the striving was to "Get closer to someone," only a single path to the desired goal would need to be found. Thus, when it comes to problem solving, avoidance goals require a very different form of analytical reasoning than approach goals. In a series of clever experiments, Coats, Janoff-Bulman, and Alpert (1996) provide evidence that goal-monitoring processes account for the differential consequences of approach versus avoidant goals. Approach goals tend to be characterized by "feature-positive searching" that is biased in favor of goal attainment, whereas avoidant goals are characterized by "feature-negative" searching. This latter type of informational search tends to be more inefficient, more effortful, and more demanding and therefore less likely to lead to successful outcomes.

A biological explanation suggests that preferences for approach versus avoidance strivings could reflect different neural processes, primarily those involving the behavioral inhibition and activation systems (Gray, 1987). Perhaps individuals preoccupied by avoidant goals have more reactive inhibition systems, and are thus preoccupied with avoiding aversive outcomes. In support of this conjecture, Emmons and McAdams (1991) found that inhibition scores from a TAT-like picture story exercise were significantly correlated with the individual's proportion of avoidant strivings. On the other hand, individuals whose striving system contains predominantly approach goals are more sensitive to rewards. Recently, Carver and White (1994) developed a questionnaire measure of Gray's behavioral activation and behavioral inhibition systems, and we have found weak positive associations between avoidance strivings and scales measuring behavioral inhibition (Emmons & Kaiser, 1996). The personal striving framework appears to be one means of accessing, albeit indirectly, these appetitive and aversive motivational systems.

The third explanation suggested itself after we (Emmons & Kaiser, 1996) examined the different patterns of appraisal for approach versus avoidance strivings. In order to determine why the avoidance strivings are so consistently related to negative outcomes, we examined the difference between how approach versus avoidance strivings are rated on the Striving Assessment Dimensions (SAS). The SAS consists of 17 appraisal dimensions that represent parameters along which people evaluate their individual goals. Compared to approach strivings, avoidance strivings tend to be rated as lower in desirability, less successfully consummated, engaged in for less autonomous or intrinsic reasons, and less likely to be supported by others in the person's social network. Deci and Ryan

(1991) have proposed that motivated behaviors vary in the degree to which they are self-determined, or autonomous, versus controlled. Acting for more autonomous reasons has been associated with more favorable outcomes in terms of academic motivation and religiosity (see Deci & Ryan, 1991, for a review). Introjected regulation (Ryan, 1995) tends to be associated with behavior being undertaken in order to avoid an undesired outcome, such as punishment. The data reported in Emmons and Kaiser (1996) indicate that subjects with a high proportion of avoidance strivings tend to be more extrinsically motivated than subjects with fewer avoidance strivings. Perhaps avoidant strivings are associated with more aversive outcomes because they reflect engaging in controlled as opposed to self-determined behavior. In their research on avoidant goals and illness described earlier, Elliot and Sheldon (1998) concluded that avoidance goals are psychological vulnerabilities that place individuals at risk for not receiving the psychological nutrients necessary for physical health. Using a vehicular analogy, the authors suggest that "approach goals are better suited for the terrain of life than are avoidance goals" (Elliot & Sheldon, 1998, p. 1294). This leads to the third and final goal orientation, the degree of self-determination.

Reasons for Striving

A third goal orientation that has been linked to well-being is derived from Deci and Ryan's (1985) self-determination theory, discussed previously. Recall that Deci and Ryan proposed that motivated behaviors vary in the degree to which they are self-determined (autonomous) versus controlled. Ryan, Sheldon, Kasser, and Deci (1996) contend that "it is only when qualities of motivation are considered that many important aspects of behavior and experience can be predicted" (p. 12). Ryan et al. developed a continuum of reasons for acting, ranging from the most extrinsic, controlling reasons to the most intrinsic, self-determined reasons, and termed this dimension "degree of self-determination." Sheldon and Kasser (1995) asked subjects to rate the degree to which they strove for each of their goals, either for internal or external reasons. Internal reasons included because the goal was personally interesting, important, and valued, or purely because of enjoyment that the striving provides. External reasons included because they felt compelled to strive by either interpersonal or intrapsychic reasons, for instance guilt or shame. Having more autonomous reasons for one's strivings was positively associated with several measures of psychological well-being, including life satisfaction, vitality, self-actualizing tendencies, and self-integration. Extrinsic orientation was related to self-reports of anxiety and depression and poorer self-integration. Degree of self-determination may be especially important for goals in the spiritual domain, as often times individuals may feel compelled to engage in religious activities without intrinsic motivation. I shall have more to say about sources of religious striving in Chapter 5.

GOAL STRUCTURE AND WELL-BEING

A third way in which to relate goals to well-being is through structural aspects of goal systems. The structural component of goal systems refers to the degree of (inter)dependence that exists between elements within a person's overall goal hierarchy. Goals may be relatively independent of each other (although complete orthogonality between goals is unlikely), instrumental for the achievement of other goals, or conflictual with respect to their mutual attainment. This systemic framework within which goals are organized emerges as a strong predictor of subjective well-being outcomes.

Conflict

A state of conflict arises when a person is prompted simultaneously by incompatible response tendencies (Janis, Mahl, Kagan, & Holt, 1969). Conflict refers to the situation in which a goal that a person wishes to accomplish interferes with the attainment of at least one other goal that the individual simultaneously wishes to accomplish. For example, the goal of trying to spend time with one's family may interfere with the goal of doing well in one's career. The debilitating effects of conflict on self-regulatory processes has been discussed in some detail by Bargh and Gollwitzer (1994), Emmons, King, and Sheldon (1993), Gollwitzer (1993), and Karoly (1993). Gollwitzer (1993) and Emmons et al. (1993) describe how individuals may resolve conflicts between competing intentions in the service of attaining valued personal goals. The inability to resolve chronic conflicts is associated with poorer well-being. In our laboratory (Emmons & King, 1988) we have found that conflict between and within personal strivings is related to measures of negative affectivity and physical symptomatology, both concurrently as well as prospectively. This aspect of goals has the most powerful influence on subjective well-being of any goal construct. The next chapter presents the evidence and discusses the relation between goal conflict and well-being.

Colby (1996) has explored the association between identity formation and goal conflict. She suggests that the process of identity development can bring previously disparate and conflicting goals into harmony.

Preliminary support for this hypothesis was found in a sample of college undergraduates (Colby, 1996). Students in the moratorium phase of identity development reported more goal conflicts compared with students who were characterized by other identity statuses. This implies that a higher-order organizational structure such as identity can result in the effective management of lower-level goal conflicts. Chapter 6 examines this idea further in the context of ultimate concerns and personality integration.

Goal Differentiation

Another structural parameter that has ramifications for well-being is the differentiation or distinctiveness that exists within one's goal system. Goal differentiation refers to the degree of interrelation that exists between individual goals in the system. A high degree of differentiation exists in systems in which goals are not highly related to each other, and are thus relatively independent. Highly differentiated persons possess a variety of strivings in a variety of domains (domain generality). A low degree of differentiation, on the other hand, is characteristic of systems in which the goals are highly related to each other, or are interdependent. Differentiation is one component of structural complexity, along with integration.

Emmons and King (1989) assessed the degree of differentiation both within and between strivings by having subjects assess the degree of (dis)similarity between all possible pairs of strivings. Subjects also indicated the number of distinct strategies they possessed for achieving each striving ("plan differentiation"). Using both an experience-sampling and daily diary methodology, striving differentiation was found to positively relate to affective reactivity. Individuals who possessed highly differentiated goal systems tended to experience more extreme affective states, and, in general, were characterized by lower levels of psychological well-being. In another study, Sheldon and Emmons (1995) found that differentiated persons tended to appraise their strivings more negatively on a number of striving dimensions. More specifically, they reported less successful attainment and lower expectancies for future attainment, and rated their strivings as more difficult than did less differentiated subjects. A similar finding was reported by Donahue, Robins, Roberts, and John (1993) who demonstrated that differentiation in the self-concept was negatively related to a variety of adjustment indicators, including emotional distress and interpersonal and occupational difficulties. Thus, taken as a whole, differentiation appears to be indicative of conflict or fragmentation within a goal system, with negative repercussions for well-being. While it is possible to have a highly elaborated and differentiated set of goals that exist in harmony with each other, in reality that appears to be a relatively rare occurrence. Intergoal relationships tend to be instrumental or conflictual. The next chapter examines the affective consequences of systemic goal conflict.

IS WELL-BEING A FUNCTION OR CONSEQUENCE OF GOAL APPRAISALS?

In the studies reviewed in this chapter, the majority of relations between goal attributes and well-being outcomes have been correlational. Such cross-sectional designs leave unanswered the question of what leads to what: Do goal appraisals generally drive well-being or do long-term levels of well-being (which are primarily determined by temperament) influence goal formation and evaluation? For example, does goal conflict lead to lower well-being or do chronic dysphoric states lead a person to appraise his or her goals more negatively, including seeing more conflict between those goals? If affect reflects the status of goal pursuits, then, logically, appraisals would precede affective reactions. But affect can also serve as an input to judgment and decision making (Schwarz, 1990). What, then, leads to what?

Myriam Mongrain and I attempted to answer this question in a mood induction study (Mongrain & Emmons, 1993). Pleasant and unpleasant moods were induced through a combination of music and autobiographical recall. No changes from baseline in goal appraisals were observed in the depressed condition. In the elated condition, subjects rated their goals less ambivalently and had a clearer idea of how to accomplish them compared to baseline. Thus, it appears that the alleviation of negative affect results in more favorable evaluations of one's goals, a finding consistent with the literature on affect and judgment (cf. Schwarz, 1990).

Another attempt to disentangle the causal direction between goal appraisals and well-being was undertaken by Brunstein (1993). In a short-term longitudinal study of young adults, he examined the interactive effects of goal commitment, attainability, and progress on well-being. They provided lists of short-term goals they intended to work on in the next few months. Measures of their well-being were taken at four points in time over a period of 14 weeks. Both affect and life satisfaction were assessed. Goal commitment was found to mediate the relationship between attainability and well-being. Specifically, students who possessed a high level of commitment and attained their goals showed positive changes in well-being over time. On the other hand, students with high levels of commitment and with fewer opportunities for goal attainment showed a decrement in well-being over time. Commitment per se was unrelated to well-being. The results supported the position that perceived progress in attainment acts to cause changes in well-being rather than vice-versa. Short-term changes in well-being appeared to be the result of shifting goal appraisals and goal outcomes.

Narrative methodologies may be a valuable means of identifying personal goals and have certain advantages over more tightly structured questionnaire measures. The intricacies of personal meaning may emerge in clearer relief when participants are allowed to tell their stories (McAdams, 1993; Singer & Salovey, 1993; Singer, 1997). Stein, Folkman, Trabasso, and Richards (1997) identified goal themes in narrative interviews of caregivers of men with AIDS. Goals and appraisals were used to prospectively predict well-being and adjustment 12 months after the death of their partner. The presence of long-term goals predicted more positive states of mind 1 year after the death, whereas an initial focus on short-term goals was a negative predictor of well-being 12 months later. This study demonstrated the importance of goal orientation on long-term subjective well-being under trying circumstances and highlighted the importance of personal goals in the coping process, a topic that I shall return to in Chapter 7.

CLINICAL APPLICATIONS

The literature reviewed in this chapter holds a number of implications for therapeutic assessment and intervention. How individuals cognitively represent their strivings may determine their motivation to seek, avoid, or stay in therapy and to make actual changes in their lives. The perceived impact that therapy may have on each striving is also likely to be influential. Identifying a client's striving structure may be quite valuable for long-term therapy. Many of the goal characteristics described in this chapter (e.g., conflict, ambivalence, avoidance) tap concerns of acute clinical significance. A number of clinically mindful investigators have described the potential benefits of incorporating a goal-based approach into the design of treatment programs (Karoly, 1991, 1993; Klinger, 1987). Karoly in particular has been vociferous in championing a goal framework for the understanding of a number of clinical and health issues. His work will be described shortly. Goals have direct applicability to a client's life, hence they often may be effective targets for change. A personal goal assessment can pinpoint problematic goal appraisals within the person's hierarchy that might be associated with psychological, somatic, or interpersonal distress. For example, an identification of goals that are overvalued, undervalued, unrealistic, conflict producing, or self-defeating would be a first step in designing an appropriate, workable intervention that would enable an individual to experience greater self-efficacy and positive states of well-being. The replacement of avoidant with approach goals or extreme high-level or low-level goals with mid-level goals may both be effective starting points for treatment.

Consider, for instance, the case of "Sissy" (a pseudonym), a 23-year-old single white female who was a participant in one of my first studies (Emmons, 1986) on personal strivings. Sissy was committed to a number of maladaptive and self-defeating strivings that appeared to be causing her a great deal of psychological distress and interpersonal conflict. She had been diagnosed as suffering from a generalized anxiety disorder, and at the time she was interviewed, she had recently experienced at least one panic attack. She was taking medication in order to reduce her excessive anxiety. Sissy's strivings are displayed in Table 3.4.

These textbook cases of irrational, unrealistic goals might have come from a client of Albert Ellis's. Some form of rational-emotive therapy might have been effective for Sissy in helping her recognize the impossibility of succeeding at these strivings. There are hints that she was aware of their unattainability. For example, after writing the striving to "Gain the approval of my father," she added in parentheses, "although I know it will never happen." In Chapter 6, I suggest an alternative approach based on Propst's (1988) religiously based cognitive therapy that appears to be effective in dealing with issues of perfectionistic striving.

Personal goals may be extremely useful as an assessment tool in counseling situations. The Striving Instrumentality Matrix (SIM) is a

TABLE 3.4. The Personal Strivings of "Sissy"

"Behave in such a way that I am accepted by everyone."
"Always be in a happy mood."
"Make people laugh."
"Be a 'mother' to everyone."
"Avoid conflict."
"Perform at perfection in my job."
"Avoid circumstances that I may fail in."
"Be accepting of everyone."
"Gain the approval of my father."
"Express my feelings toward my boyfriend."
"Do too much in too little time."
"Appear 'together' all of the time."
"Live an independent lifestyle."
"Plan ahead in as many situations as I can."
"Get others to agree with my reasoning related to a decision I've made."

useful way of assessing the degree of self-perceived conflict between one's strivings. I have also found that objective raters are reasonably accurate at judging the degree of conflict between a target individual's strivings. Since conflict is often a culprit in personal and interpersonal difficulties, the SIM would appear to possess a great deal of applicability. Individuals who have completed the SIM have remarked that it was extremely useful to have thought about their strivings in this way and that it helped them identify problem areas in their life to focus on. I explore some specific examples in the next chapter and in Chapter 6.

The personal goals of young men and women seeking counseling was the focus of a study by Salmela-Aro (1992). Her research, framed within a larger context of understanding psychosocial factors involved in the transition to adulthood, compared the personal goals (or projects) of clients with two nonclinical samples. The client group was characterized by a pattern of maladaptive goal striving. Not only were their projects more self-focused compared to nonclinical samples, their goals were also more unrealistic, and they were less likely to have reported making satisfactory progress. Salmela-Aro suggested that an effective therapeutic strategy would be to assist clients in lowering attainment standards and breaking down broad goals into manageable, mid-level goals. In a study of "social dropouts" (Salmela-Aro, Nurmi, & Ruotsalainen, 1995), young persons with unstable employment histories had lower expectancies for goal accomplishment compared to a control group and were more likely to attribute success at their goals to external, uncontrollable forces as opposed to internal, controllable factors. Goal interventions might also be effective here.

Goal Cognitions as a Tool in Clinical Assessment

In a number of recent publications in the 1990s, clinical psychologist Paul Karoly has argued that goals may take on an acute clinical significance and therefore are relevant to a variety of concerns in a clinical context. An impressive research program by Karoly and his associates has documented that goals are workable clinical units for assessment and therapy for both mental and physical health outcomes (Karoly, 1991, 1993; Lecci, Karoly, Ruehlman, & Lanyon, 1996; Karoly & McKeeman, 1991). Employing a self-regulatory framework, Karoly has developed the Goal Systems Assessment Battery (GSAB), which assesses a variety of mechanisms related to goal setting and progress evaluation. Issues in the setting, selection, and scheduling of goals (collectively known as goal cognitions) have been found to be predictive of chronic pain (Affleck et al., 1998; Karoly & Ruehlman, 1996), hypochondriacal tendencies (Lecci et al., 1996), cessation of smoking (Karoly & McKeeman,

1991), medical compliance (Karoly, 1991; Karoly & Bay, 1990) and the distinction between the clinical states of depression and anxiety (Lecci, Karoly, Briggs, & Kuhn, 1994). Affleck et al. (1998) state that goal striving is a key cognitive-motivational construct for chronic pain experience, in that chronic pain patients contextualize their symptoms with respect to their impact on valued goals. Karoly provides considerable evidence that goal variables are moderators (1) of the relation between life stress and illness, (2) between attitudes and self-protective actions, and (3) between chronic illness states and subjective health outcomes. As such, the motivational perspective centered around personal goals has considerable value for addressing multiple problems in clinical assessment and treatment.

The venues in which the goal framework may ultimately prove most useful to clinical cases are too numerous to be fully dealt with in all of their complexity in this book. This section of the chapter has briefly considered some potential applications. Underscoring the sentiments presented at the outset of Chapter 2 on the centrality of goals in human lives, the goal construct does appear to be a powerful unit of analysis for understanding issues central to human adaptation, and is relevant to both optimal as well as to suboptimal functioning.

CHAPTER FOUR

Goal Conflict and Personality Fragmentation

*I*n a perfect world, our goal pursuits would run smoothly. We would have a clear idea of what we needed to accomplish, opportunities for attainment would abound, and significant others would readily support our most cherished ambitions. But we do not live in a perfect world. Ambitions are frustrated. Our goals are not always met with open arms by others. Opportunities to make progress may be few and far between. Perhaps the most formidable obstacle we face comes not from the outside, but from within. Our own goals may be in competition with each other.

Goal conflicts are part of the human experience. When there are choices to be made or decisions to be reached, competing desires are frequently involved. We desire many things in life—we want affection from loved ones, recognition from our peers, a comfortable lifestyle. Other desires may keep us from achieving all that we want. We want to maintain our independence from others, we want to avoid calling attention to ourselves, we want to live a simple and frugal life. We wish to spend time with our family, but we wish to advance in our career. We want to take risks, but we want to be secure. People handle conflict differently, one person may be immobilized by what seems to be the most trivial conflict, while the next person seems to move effortlessly through life, seemingly free of conflict. Research has confirmed that conflict is a major source of suffering and misery in people's lives. Conflicting motives systems are a source of self-regulatory failure. Poorly handled, chronic conflicts are at the root of many physical illnesses and poor mental and emotional health. Depression, anxiety, ulcers, and heart disease have all been associated with the inner psychological turmoil that surrounds unresolved conflicts. Conflict appears to be the "Achilles heel" of goal striving.

Conflict is a fascinating topic. It is one of the thorniest in the psychological literature, and one of the most difficult to study empirically. One of the reasons why I was initially attracted to the concept of goals as a theoretical construct in personality psychology was because of its potential in elucidating the causes and consequences of intrapsychic conflicts. The internal battles that all of us struggle with from time to time (some of us chronically so) have a way of becoming perpetual sources of misery and suffering. All the more vital, then, to construct relatively permanent solutions to conflicting motivations. Toward the end of this chapter, I briefly comment on modes of conflict resolution, and then return to this topic in Chapter 6 in the context of personality integration.

Although conflict is ubiquitous in everyday life and in a wealth of theoretical and clinical writings, conflict as a research topic is relatively recent. In 1985, Pervin concluded his chapter in the *Annual Review of Psychology* by stating that "I am struck by the power of conflicting motivations in my patients and the absence of such phenomena in the literature" (p. 105). Since Pervin's charge, a scattering of research on conflict has appeared in the empirical literature. My goal in this chapter is to review research and theory on the concept of psychological conflict, with an emphasis on the role of conflict in both psychological and physical well-being. Evidence is reviewed indicating that the failure to control conflict results in psychological and physical distress, ruminative cognitions, and less effective regulation of behavior.

Personal goals serve as an ideal vehicle for examining intrapsychic conflict since everyday decisional conflicts often revolve around fundamental values, goals, and desires. In their classic volume on personality and society, Kluckhohn and Murray (1953) commented that "the most difficult and painful function of personality [is] that of accommodating its expressions, needs, choice of goal-objects, methods, and time-programs to the patterns that are conventionally sanctioned by society" (p. 19). This comment suggests that action can be seen as a compromise between the broad range of an individual's needs and situational and self-imposed constraints. Behavioral impulses must be controlled or inhibited when they are at odds with a person's overarching goals and values or with societal constraints. We cannot have or do all that we desire because often our desires themselves are mutually exclusive. At the same time, conflict can be both beneficial and detrimental to well-being. It may be in one's best interest to refrain from angry impulses to one's boss, for instance, or to forgo the short-term thrill of a romantic affair in the interest of a committed relationship. At the same time, chronic inhibition of desires due to conflict is associated with ruminative cognitions, psychological distress, and physical illness (Emmons & King, 1988; Pennebaker, 1989). Conflictual material about which a person attempts to avoid thinking is likely to intrude into consciousness. Thus, gaining control over conflicting motivations is a primary goal of individual psychotherapy and spiritual practices.

THEORETICAL PERSPECTIVES ON CONFLICT

A number of theoretical perspectives have over the years employed the concept of conflict between motivational tendencies as a means to better understand and explain human personality and psychopathology. Theorists and researchers beginning with Freud have stressed the necessity of avoiding inner conflict by maintaining consistency and harmony among aspects of the psyche, and the injurious consequences of failing to do so. McReynolds (1990) provides a historical overview of the construct from the early Greeks to modern time. The concept of conflict has been of central concern in psychodynamic, behavioral, and cognitive formulations (see Emmons et al., 1993 and Epstein, 1982, for reviews). In control theory language, for example, conflict is the inability to match two or more reference values simultaneously (Carver & Scheier, 1998). Within these various theoretical perspectives, a number of terms have been used to describe oppositional tendencies within the mind. These include discrepancies, disregulations, disconnections, contradictions, incongruities, incompatibilities, imbalances, and discontinuities. Regardless of terminological differences, these perspectives are all dealing with internal incompatibilities—that is, conflict.

Conflicts are problem situations that involve two competing and mutually exclusive alternative resolutions (McReynolds, 1990). A good all-purpose definition is provided by Heitler (1990): "Conflict is a situation in which seemingly incompatible elements exert force in opposing or divergent directions" (p. 5). Conflicts have a discernible grammar— they are expressed as oppositional statements ("I want to write this book but I also want to play golf"). A conflict may involve opposing feelings toward the same object, a condition normally referred to as "ambivalence." Meehl (1964) defined intense ambivalence as "the existence of simultaneous or rapidly interchangeable positive and negative feelings toward the same object or activity, with the added proviso that both the positive and negative feelings be strong" (p. 10). Clearly, this definition conjures up a conflict situation. Ambivalence can also be thought of as an approach–avoidance conflict—wanting but at the same time not wanting the same goal object. For example, a person may be ambivalent about the goal to "Express my true feelings" because of the potential negative consequences that such free expression might entail. In addition, an individual may be ambivalent about the goal to "Finish my dissertation as soon as possible" not because the end is viewed as potentially negative, but because the process of achieving the goal may seem unusually daunting. The second use of the term conflict refers to the situation in which a goal that a person wishes to accomplish interferes with the attainment of at least one other goal that the individual simultaneously wishes to accomplish. For example, the goal of trying to "Spend time with my family" may interfere with the goal of trying to "Do well in my career." Epstein (1982) described several forms of conceptual conflict that may be experienced as stressful. He listed five basic sources of conceptual incompatibility that reflect various types of conflict:

> (a) incompatibilities between an individual's beliefs and the occurrence of events inconsistent with those beliefs, (b) incompatibilities between an individual's ideal self and actual self, (c) incompatibilities between differing beliefs or values of which the individual is aware, (d) incompatibilities between beliefs in what is and what should be or should have been, and (e) incompatibilities between beliefs at different levels of awareness. (p. 63)

Wilensky (1983) discussed the various types of conflict that can occur between goals at both an intrapersonal and interpersonal level. At the intrapersonal level, goals may be in opposition to each other, where the pursuit of one interferes with the pursuit of another. Similarly, at the interpersonal level, the goals of two or more individuals may be in competition. Wilensky's thorough analysis includes a discussion of the various classes of reasons why goals can come into conflict, and offers suggestions as to how such conflicts might be resolved. The debilitating effects of conflict on psychological well-being and physical health have been well-documented (see Emmons et al., 1993, for a review). The inability to resolve chronic conflicts is associated with poorer mental health, risk for physical illness, and relationship dissatisfaction. Lazarus (1991) cogently summarizes the conflict–distress link in the following: "Whereas integration is tantamount to mental health, disconnection among the constructs of the mind is tantamount to psychopathology, dysfunction, and distress. The three constructs of the mind—cognition, emotion, and motivation—should generally be compatible, ideally in harmony; the mind as a system must also be in reasonable touch with environmental conditions; and actions should flow from this harmony" (pp. 460–461).

Another term that is used to portray a situation of conflict is *alienation*. According to Finger (1997), alienation is "a pervasive condition in which elements that belong together, which should be supporting and sustaining each other and which ultimately cannot survive apart, are profoundly estranged and hostile" (p. 13). The term is more often used in theological (being alienated from God) and sociological contexts (alienation from society) than in the psychological community, though it is not unfamiliar in existential approaches to psychotherapy. In this latter case it generally denotes a sense of meaninglessness and apathy more so than internal division. Though it may accurately describe the psychological experience of conflicted individuals, because of its surplus meaning I will generally avoid the use of it in this chapter.

Conflict and the Fragmented Self

Lifton (1993) has described the current historical period as the "age of fragmentation." Named after the Greek god Proteus, Lifton describes the "protean self," the prototypical character style of our time. Lacking a stable coherent core, the protean self is in continuous flux, without integrity or mooring, in short, a fragmented, divided self: "The fragmented self is radically bereft of coherence and continuity, an extreme expression of dissociation" (Lifton, 1993, p. 202). When I use the term "fragmentation," I will do so in a much more circumscribed way than does Lifton. By fragmentation I mean simply a self that is characterized by a high degree of systemic goal conflict, where the person's various long-term aims are essentially incompatible. He or she may or may not be fully aware of these incompatibilities and yet may feel a strong sense of alienation or internal separation. I am not dealing with the more extreme forms of fragmentation that Lifton describes in his book, which might be seen in the clinically diagnosable disorders of multiple or borderline personality, or the schizophrenias. Paradoxically, consciously experienced, garden-variety fragmentation may be more psychologically distressing than the severer forms of fragmentation, in which protective structures have developed.

MEASURING GOAL CONFLICT

People vary greatly in their subjective experience of conflict. Whereas one person might be paralyzed by even the slightest decisional conflict, another may live a life totally free from regrets and second guessing. Evidence from various clinical and nonclinical populations suggests that individual differences do exist in the subjective experience of conflict (King & Emmons, 1990; Sincoff, 1990). To assess individual differences in conflict, we (Emmons & King, 1988) have employed a number of different procedures. We begin with the identification of goals that the person is currently working on. In the personal striving framework (see Chapter 2), subjects begin by completing a series of 15 open-ended statements, the stem of which is "I typically try to _____." Following generation of the strivings, subjects complete a 15 × 15 matrix (striving instrumentality matrix [SIM]), in which the rows and columns consist of the person's strivings. The degree of facilitation or hindrance between each pair of strivings is rated until the entire matrix is filled out by the subject. Each goal is in effect rated twice, in terms of the effect that it has on other goals and the effect that other goals have on it. For the matrix as a whole, the average amount of conflict or instrumentality in the person's goal system is determined and is used as a variable in between-subject analyses. This method for measuring conflict has proven useful in studies described later in this chapter. Cox and Klinger (1988) have demonstrated the applicability of the SIM for motivational counseling with alcoholics, and Karoly (1991) has described its potential for health issues. Of course, ours is only one approach among many that are feasible. Other methods for assessing goal conflicts are described in Lauterbach (1990) and McReynolds (1990). Examples of conflicting striving pairs are shown in Table 4.1.

Ambivalence over goal strivings can be assessed by asking subjects the degree of unhappiness they would experience upon successful consummation of the striving (after Klinger, 1987). The reliability of this single-item measure is enhanced by aggregating across all of the subject's goal strivings. Various other probes may be used to measure within-goal conflict, such as having subjects rate the amount of relief experienced upon the abandonment of a goal, and distinguishing between ambivalence in working toward the goal versus ambivalence felt after the goal is

TABLE 4.1. Examples of Strivings Rated as Conflicting

"Ease others' lives" versus "Make myself happy"
"Be sincere and straightforward" versus "Control my stress"
"Keep an ongoing relationship with my family" versus "Avoid getting into arguments"
"Succeed in school" versus "Please myself"
"Be competent in my work" versus "Spend time with family and friends"
"Find solitude" versus "Be supportive of family and friends"
"Live a 'godly' life" versus "Make people like me"
"Be assertive" versus "Say only what is necessary"
"Be very self-critical" versus "Realize my limitations"
"Influence nonbelievers toward faith" versus "Not live by others' approval"
"Be spiritually strong" versus "Make myself physically attractive"
"Be a seeker of the truth" versus "Do well in school"

achieved. Karoly (1991) has asked subjects to indicate the degree to which the goal is in their best interest; we have found that this item correlates positively with other striving ambivalence items.

Goal Conflict and Physical Health

Conflicts are sources of stress. As such, they increase an organism's potential for stress-induced disease. Chronic conflicting motivations are associated with decrements in physical functioning. The links between conflict, physiological processes, and disease outcomes have been demonstrated in both human and nonhuman populations. Nearly a half-century ago, Alexander (1950) presented a psychosomatic theory in which specific unconscious conflicts rooted in childhood experiences were believed to produce specific physical diseases. While specificity theory paid insufficient attention to plausible mechanisms by which conflict can lead to disease, current work has begun to explore these possible pathways. In addition, current work employs a different conceptualization of conflict. Nevertheless, many of these conflict models have their impetus in Alexander's formulations.

Sawrey and Weisz (1956) produced gastric ulcers in rats by creating an approach–avoidance conflict. Food and water were obtainable only if rats crossed an electrified grid floor. This study was notable because it was the first to demonstrate that gastric ulcers could be produced without a direct physiological manipulation. The authors concluded that stress resulting from the chronic conflict situation was the crucial factor in ulcer production. Lawler, Barker, Hubbard, and Allen (1980) demonstrated that compared to controls, rats subjected to approach–avoidance conflict developed tonic levels of systolic high blood pressure in the hypertensive range.

The relationship between conflict and physiological arousal has also been demonstrated in humans. Mann, Janis, and Chaplin (1969) showed that decisional conflict is related to increased heart rate and skin conductance responding during a decision-making experiment. In their classic work, Janis and Mann (1977) review evidence that decision making is stressful. The degree of stress is directly related to the magnitude of the consequences of the decision, particularly the perceived magnitude of the losses associated with whatever choice is made (Janis & Mann, 1977). Janis and Mann (1977) observe that a number of American presidents have suffered deleterious physical effects when preoccupied with critical decisional conflicts, such as whether or not to enter war or to resign from office in the face of scandal.

McClelland (1989) has investigated conflict over expressing power, as reflected in a high degree of power motivation coupled with a tendency to inhibit overt power actions (activity inhibition). This motive pattern has been linked with chronic high blood pressure, lower immunocompetence levels, and subsequent susceptibility to stress-related illnesses.

In addition to conflict in motivational systems, connections between conflict and illness have been addressed through more cognitive perspectives as well. Conflicting beliefs play a major role in Kreitler and Kreitler's (1991) cognitive orientation (CO) theory of physical illness. CO theory is too detailed to permit a lengthy treatment here, but, briefly, the Kreitlers' primary interest has been in specifying beliefs and intents underlying health-related behaviors. Relevant to this theory is a study by Kreitler and Chemerinski (1988), who found that a variety of conflicts differentiated between obese and nonobese individuals. These included conflicts over interpersonal relations and conflicts over work and career aims (e.g., achievement vs. fear of failure). Overeating in obese individuals may be a response to the stress associated with the conflicts from which these individuals suffer.

Dixon and Dixon (1991) examined value and role conflicts in professional women. A survey to assess the degree of perceived tension or competition between different life domains (family, work, education) was administered to 300 women between 50 and 70 years of age with postgraduate degrees in either nursing or in other health fields. High scores on the "Career–Life Balance Inventory" indicated that they recognized tension in integrating career aspirations with other aspects of life. They found that tension between career involvements and interpersonal commitments successfully discriminated women with self-reported cardiovascular disease (who had high levels of conflict) from women with self-reported cancer (who reported low levels of conflict). Those in the cardiovascular group reported the most difficulties in balancing their careers with other aspects of their lives. The retrospective design of this study requires that the results be interpreted cautiously. However, they do suggest the possibility that chronic conflict may be a potential risk factor in the development and/or exacerbation of cardiac symptomatology, most likely through physiological mechanisms of chronic sympathetic reactivity found in the animal studies described earlier.

Ewart (1991) developed a theoretical model linking interpersonal goal congruence and other goal mechanisms to health outcomes, health protective behaviors, and coping with acute myocardial infarction. He also found (Ewart, 1994) that relative to a group whose strivings were primarily concerned with personal growth, subjects whose primary goals entailed trying to *change someone else* exhibited larger blood pressure increases when discussing a personal problem. This is the only study with which I am familiar that has examined striving content as a predictor of cardiovascular reactivity. Goal system variables (in this case goal content) may thus be a risk factor for cardiovascular disease through persisting high blood pressure. This finding is reminiscent of McClelland's (1989) work cited earlier on power motivation and chronic hypertension.

Karoly and McKeeman (1991) asked chronic smokers to rate the degree to which each of their personal goals interfered with the goal of quitting smoking. They also assessed conflict in the form of hindrance from significant others. Participants were divided into three groups: smokers, relapsers, and quitters. Successful quitters were less likely to perceive conflicts between quitting smoking and other goals of theirs, and were less likely to perceive hindrance from others in their goal to quit smoking. Relapsers and smokers did not differ from each other on intergoal conflict or interpersonal hindrance. This interesting study demonstrated that conflicting motive systems can be a source of self-regulatory failure.

In what are now a classic series of studies, as reviewed by Pennebaker (1990), these studies have shown that individuals who inhibit their desire to confide in others about traumatic life events but still think about them are more likely to develop physical illnesses, such as flus, ulcers, and respiratory infections. Inhibition is also related to lower immunocompetence (Pennebaker, Kiecolt-Glaser, & Glaser, 1989). A desire to confide, coupled with a fear of confiding (i.e., conflict) results in increased rumination, chronic autonomic arousal, and eventual physiological distress. Other evidence suggests that the related conflictual personality styles of repressive-defensiveness and the inability to express intense negative emotion are linked to the development and progression of a variety of serious illnesses, including cancer and essential hypertension (Friedman & Booth-Kewley, 1987).

In our laboratory we have found that conflict between and within personal strivings is related to measures of negative affectivity and physical symptomatology, both concurrently as well as prospectively (Emmons & King, 1988). Conflict (between goals) and ambivalence (approach–avoidance conflict) are associated with a variety of physical symptoms as well as an increase in health center visits and actual number of distinct illness diagnosed there during a 1-year follow-up (Emmons & King, 1988). Interpersonal goal conflict is also related to lower psychological well-being and to physical illness (King & Emmons, 1991). Emmons and King (1988) found that individuals did tend to inhibit behavior over conflictful strivings yet tended to spend time thinking about these same conflictful goals. High levels of rumination and inhibition were associated with low levels of psychological and physical well-being, which is consistent with Pennebaker's "active inhibition" model. Based on our results linking conflict to inhibition and rumination, as well as the accumulating evidence suggestive of the negative health effects of inhibition, Emmons and King (1988) proposed that any desire (or goal) to act that is coupled with a desire (or goal) to inhibit action is stressful and, if chronic and unintegrated, is likely to induce aversive psychological and physical states. Thus, a number of studies have demonstrated relations between chronic psychological conflict and autonomic nervous system functioning, thereby strengthening the case for conflict as a precursor to physical illness. It has become evident that an inability to control conflict is a source of stress (Epstein, 1982), and, as such, sets into motion pathogenic processes increasing illness risk over time.

The Value of a Strivings Perspective

Conflicts among personal strivings may have particularly important ramifications for the individual, since they reflect chronic conflict at levels higher in the motivational hierarchy, more central to the self-concept. Strivings provide information on not only what a person is trying to do, but also on who a person is trying to be. Striving conflict may reflect an underlying clash of basic values, not just a problem of resisting stray impulses or scheduling competing intentions efficiently. To the extent that the strivings in conflict involve deeper values rather than well-defined behavioral objectives, conflict may become more problematic. For example, one subject rated the strivings of trying to "Appear more intelligent than I am" and trying to "Always present myself in an honest light" as being in conflict. The profound duality of purpose implied by these two strivings indicates a problem not likely to be resolved by self-distraction. Because higher levels within a hierarchical control system (Carver & Scheier, 1998; Powers, 1973) tend to be more self-definitional, conflict between high-level strivings may tend to strain or even overwhelm action systems, resulting in persistent negative affect. This suggestion is supported by Emmons's (1992) finding that people with high-level strivings tend to experience more conflict and more negative affect, particularly depression.

Another reason why conflict between high-level goals may be less likely to be ameliorated is that high-level goals are less likely to become conscious in the course of everyday behavior. High-level strivings, which tend to be self-defining, value-laden motivational tendencies, are less likely to become manifest as conscious intentions while the person behaves, compared to low-level intentions such as "Mowing the lawn this afternoon." Only if the person becomes alert to the influence of both conflicting strivings within a given situation (e.g., "Wanting this person to think I'm smart" and "Not being a phony") is he or she in a position to use active information-processing strategies to inhibit one of them. In order to employ these strategies, however, the person must be able to make a conscious commitment to one of the two competing values. Even if he or she does manage to choose and promote one of the two strivings, these information-processing strategies are likely to fail in the long run; a transient impulse will eventually go away, but a suppressed basic motive probably will not.

Some conflicts may be the result of clashes between high- and low-level intentions, or between more abstract versus more concrete goals. In Chapter 3, I reviewed Kasser's research program; he has found (Kasser & Ryan, 1993, 1996) that the intrinsic goals of self-acceptance and community altruism tend to promote happiness, while the extrinsic concerns of making money and personal appearance appear to detract from happiness. With respect to spiritual goals, one might also predict the potential for conflict with more material goals or "passions of the flesh." Societal factors play a major role in producing the conditions where contradictions or incompatibilities between various types of pursuits become magnified. For instance, in a culture where the good life is defined in terms of health, wealth, and status, little support is given to spiritual pursuits. In a later chapter, I look at how spiritual goals might be involved in the integration of the self. What can foster inner congruence can also offer a compelling solution to Lifton's (1993) protean self. Chapter 6 considers the valuable role that spirituality may play in the long-term resolution of conflict and subsequent personality integration, enabling the person to go from "goal to whole."

Goal Conflict and Subjective Well-Being

Historically, the presence of chronic conflicts been linked with a multitude of negative affective states and processes, including tension, uncertainty, confusion, and vacillation (Miller, 1959) as well as anxiety, depression, hostility, delusions, and hallucinations (Powers, 1973). In fact, Powers (1973) contended that "conflict represents the most serious kind of malfunction of the brain short of physical damage" (p. 253). Although perhaps not so dramatic as Powers's conclusion, empirical evidence is continually accruing in support of the notion that conflict is stressful and is associated with both psychological and physical ill-being. Palys and Little (1983) found that conflict between personal goal projects was associated with low life satisfaction. Exploring conflict between motives rather than goals, Zeldow, Daugherty, and McAdams (1988) found that high levels of intimacy and power motivation within the same person (presumably indicating motivational conflict) was related to high levels of depression and neuroticism and with low levels of self-esteem and extraversion. Perring, Oatley, and Smith (1988) related conflict between daily plans and activities to indices of emotional health. These authors distinguished between implicit and explicit conflict, a distinction that is roughly equivalent to the one made earlier between ambivalence within a goal and conflict between goals. Conflict scores were related to high levels of anxiety, depression, and social dysfunction, with the effects for explicit conflict being generally larger than those for the implicit form of conflict. Lauterbach (1975, 1990) has also extensively studied the relation between emotion and intrapersonal conflict. Defining conflict in terms of inconsistencies and contradictions amongst attitudes, beliefs, and values, he has found strong concurrent relations between conflict and depression, tension, and fatigue. Lauterbach (1975) also presented evidence that changes in naturally occurring conflict predicted changes in mood over a 5-month period.

A somewhat different approach to studying the conflict–distress link is through Higgins's (1987) self-concept discrepancy theory. According to this theory, the incompatibility of two self-conceptions leads to characteristic negative emotional states, such as sadness, anxiety, and depression. Conflict among goals are roughly equivalent to "contradictions among one's self-perceived attributes" in Higgins's terminology. It is conceivable that the objectives that a person is trying to accomplish could result from the wishes of others, thereby representing "oughts." For example, the goal trying to "Make life easier for my parents" could be the result of perceived familial obligations and could come into conflict with a self-generated striving like trying to "Have as much fun as possible." This goal situation would be an instance of an actual/own:ought/other discrepancy that is predicted to produce anxiety-related emotions, according to self-discrepancy theory. Strauman, Lemieux, and Coe (1991) have demonstrated that the activation of self-discrepancies is associated with a decrease in natural killer (NK) cell activity, thus providing evidence of a possible mechanism linking conflict with disease.

Lecci, Okun, and Karoly (1994) examined regrets as psychological conflicts. Regrets are personal goals set earlier in life but never achieved. What makes them regrets is that the person wishes he or she had pursued the goal. Regrets were found to be significant predictors of life satisfaction and depression, above and beyond the effects of goals. Depression was associated with feelings of disappointment from not having pursued the goal. The authors suggest that the subjective awareness of conflict might be adaptive. If a person can persuade himself or herself that a goal was not pursued because it conflicted with a more valuable goal, psychological distress might be avoided. Thus, it appears that there might be some conditions under which perceived conflict might facilitate emotional health.

AMBIVALENCE OVER EXPRESSING EMOTION

In the work described up to this point, conflict is typically treated in a global form, with greater conflict believed to produce greater levels of distress. No distinctions are made in the content of conflict. Yet some types of goals may be more likely to engender conflict and ambivalence than others. A content analysis of the types of strivings that individuals rated high in ambivalence in earlier research (Emmons & King, 1988) revealed a theme of conflict over expressing emotion. Given our culture's general emphasis on the containment of emotional expression coupled with a natural tendency to seek expression it is not surprising that individuals become ambivalent over emotional expression. Goals about emotional expression provide a pointed demonstration of the translation of cultural ambivalence into individual lives. For example, rated high in ambivalence were strivings such as trying to "Keep my anger under control," "Express myself honestly," "Control my temper," "Always appear cool," "Not let my emotions take over," "Always wear a smile on my face," "Be honest and open about my feelings," and "Let my anger out before it all builds up inside me." These goals illustrate the belief that emotion should be honestly expressed but also that expression implies vulnerability.

Emotions and goals share a natural relationship. Emotions serve as a gauge of our progress in our goal pursuits. We feel anger, joy, envy, and so on, in response to the frustration or fulfillment of our desires. Not only do emotions and emotional expression arise out of goals, emotion and expression can be used in the service of goals as well.

That individuals are ambivalent about emotional expression would also appear to be justified to some extent by research showing emotional expression to be related to both positive and negative psychological, physical, and interpersonal functioning (King & Emmons, 1991). The double-edged sword of emotional expression in the realm of individual functioning prompted the development of the construct of ambivalence over emotional expression. One problem in research on the relation between emotional expression and health is that because only overt styles of expression are measured, comfortable inexpressive individuals cannot be distinguished from individuals who are, in fact, tense, inhibited, and potentially at risk for a number of adverse consequences. Originating in previously described work on goal conflict (Emmons & King, 1988), conflict over emotional expression refers to an individual's comfort within his or her typical style of emotional expression. King and Emmons (1990) have suggested that inhibition of emotional expression might be understood as a result of an individual's competing desires to express and not to express emotions. Thus, inexpressiveness that may be pathogenic is distinguished from "comfortable" inexpressiveness by the conflict dynamic that exists beneath the overt expressiveness style. Conflict is presented as the key to the pathogenic quality of emotional control.

Ambivalence over emotional expression refers to the experience of conflict over one's typical expressiveness style, regardless of the style itself. Individuals may be ambivalent over the expression of emotion as well as the lack of expression. For example, an individual may wish he or she could exert more control over his or her spontaneous emotional display. In addition, an individual may feel conflict over expressing emotion because, although he or she is comfortable as an inexpressive person, social pressure to be more expressive and "open up" is brought to bear. Individuals may experience conflict over the expression of positive or negative emotions.

In order to do research on ambivalence over emotional expression, it was essential to have a psychometrically sound instrument for assessing it. With this in mind, we (King & Emmons, 1990) developed a questionnaire designed to tap individual differences in ambivalence (Ambivalence Over Expressing Emotion Questionnaire [AEQ]; see items in Table 4.2). Goals that pertained to emotional expression were culled from the striving lists of several hundred subjects and compiled into a list. This list was used as a basis for the generation of items in the AEQ. The strivings were reworded in order to address their potentially ambiv-

TABLE 4.2. The Ambivalence Over Expressing Emotion Questionnaire

Below and on the next page are statements that refer to typically occurring emotional reactions. The statements may consist of two thoughts. Carefully read the statement as a whole before deciding how characteristic it is of you. For example, consider the item: "I try to honestly criticize others for their own good, but I worry that they may get angry with me if I do so." You would give this item a high rating if and only if you BOTH try honestly to criticize others AND worry about their getting angry. If you simply try to criticize others and you don't worry about their anger, or if you don't try to criticize others at all, then you would rate this item lower. It is important to consider the complete thoughts being expressed before you respond.

1. I want to express my emotions honestly but I am afraid that it may cause me embarrassment or hurt.
2. I try to control my jealousy concerning my partner even though I want to let him or her know I'm hurting.

3. I make an effort to control my temper at all times even though I'd like to act on these feelings at times.

4. I try to avoid sulking even when I feel like it.

5. When I am really proud of something I accomplish I want to tell someone, but I fear I would be thought of as conceited.

6. I would like to express my affection more physically but I am afraid others will get the wrong impression.

7. I try not worry others, even though sometimes they should know the truth.

8. Often I'd like to show others how I feel, but something seems to be holding me back.

9. I strive to keep a smile on my face in order to convince others I am happier than I really am.

10. I try to keep my deepest fears and feelings hidden, but at times I'd like to open up to others.

11. I'd like to talk about my problems with others, but at times I just can't.

12. When someone bothers me, I try to appear indifferent even though I'd like to tell him or her how I feel.

13. I try to refrain from getting angry at my parents even though I want to at times.

14. I try to show people I love them, although at times I am afraid that it may make me appear weak or too sensitive.

15. I try to apologize when I have done something wrong but I worry that I will be perceived as incompetent.

16. I think about acting out when I am angry but I try not to.

17. Often I find that I am not able to tell others how much they really mean to me.

18. I want to tell someone when I love him or her, but it is difficult to find the right words.

19. I would like to express my disappointment when things don't go as well as planned, but I don't want to appear vulnerable.

20. I can recall a time when I wished I had told someone how much I really cared for him or her.

21. I try to hide my negative feelings around others, even though I am not being fair to those close to me.

22. I would like to be more spontaneous in my emotional reactions but I just can't seem to do it.

23. I try to suppress my anger, but I would like other people to know how I feel.

24. It is hard to find the right words to indicate to others what I am really feeling.

25. I worry that if I express negative emotions such as fear or anger, other people will not approve of me.

26. I feel guilty after I have expressed anger to someone.

27. I often cannot bring myself to express what I am really feeling.

28. After I express anger at someone, it bothers me for a long time.

alent character. For instance, the striving "I typically strive to express my emotions honestly" became "I want to express my emotions honestly but I am afraid that it may cause me embarrassment or hurt." Starting with 48 items, traditional psychometric procedures such as item analyses, reliability analyses, and factor analyses were applied to the scale. Weak items, identified by low item–total correlations and high correlations with a social desirability index were eliminated, resulting in a psychometrically sound 28-item measure that has now been used by a number of different investigators in several studies.

A number of studies have now documented that an internal struggle over expressiveness ultimately creates subjective distress, an increased risk for physical symptoms, and maladaptive transactions with the interpersonal environment. Although it has been found to relate negatively to emotional expressiveness, conflict over emotional expression, measured via this questionnaire, has been distinguished from simple inexpressiveness in studies demonstrating that ambivalence over emotional expression is related to depression, anxiety, and guilt, as well as other measures of distress, and to symptom reports, controlling for self-reported expressiveness (King & Emmons, 1990). Thus, whether the ambivalent individual is expressive or not, he or she may experience the distress associated with the underlying conflict dynamic. Importantly, these relations between distress, symptoms, and ambivalence over expression persisted even when controlling for overall negative affectivity, a procedure that has become commonplace in studies of emotional well-being and personality.

In research on married couples, ambivalence over emotional expression was related not only to individuals' experienced distress but also to the ambivalent individuals' spouses' symptomatology and alcohol consumption (King & Emmons, 1991). Husbands' ambivalence over emotional expression was negatively related to both husbands' and wives' marital satisfaction (King, 1993). In another study (Mongrain & Emmons, 1997), ambivalence was associated with poor conflict resolution skills within romantic relationships, suggesting another deficit in interpersonal functioning associated with ambivalence over emotional expression.

These results support the contention that emotional expression may be seen as a motivated behavior. In addition, results thus far support the contention that overt expressiveness styles are less directly related to well-being than is conflict over expression. Once again, the conflict that may underlie individuals' control efforts is found to play an important role in whether control exerts adverse effects.

The place of ambivalence over emotional expression in a more general model of inhibition has been addressed (King, Emmons, & Woodley, 1992). Factor-analytic results of a number of measures of inhibition and ruminative thinking indicated that conflict over emotional expression involves both the control of emotion and rumination. These findings seem to indicated that the AEQ represents a measure of a potentially pathogenic inhibitory process. Preliminary evidence also suggests that the AEQ is more predictive of psychological than physical health.

The Social Context of Emotional Ambivalence

An interesting implication suggested by research in the area of ambivalence over emotional expression is the possibility of social sources of ambivalence. Some theories imply that it would be more detrimental for an individual to be forced by social pressure to forsake a personally consistent inexpressive style than to be allowed to be inexpressive. In addition, it may be that individuals who would be expressive develop an expressive style in response to negative interpersonal interactions. Personality processes have been conceived as internalized representations of interpersonal patterns (Westen, 1992).

Emmons and Colby (1995) presented a model in which emotional conflict, including ambivalence over expressing emotion and fear of intimacy (Descutner & Thelen, 1991), is linked with distress via interpersonal pathways. This model attempts to link intrapsychic conflict with its interpersonal consequences. Specifically, a reduction in social support stemming from conflicted individuals' failure to solicit and utilize available aid was shown to mediate the relationship between conflict and well-being. Perceived social support did in fact mediate the relation between emotional conflict and well-being. Subjects answered questionnaire measures of emotional ambivalence, fear of intimacy, repressive-defensiveness, social support, and well-being. These self-report measures were included in a larger packet of questionnaires. Subjects then completed daily mood and experience forms for 21 consecutive days. In these daily forms subjects indicated, among other things, how they coped with a particular personal problem that day, and the emotions experienced during the day. Observer reports of social support provided and requested were obtained from subject's peers, relatives, and others. Conscious emotional conflict (i.e., ambivalence over expressing emotion, and fear of intimacy) was associated with lower perceived support and increased use of avoidant coping strategies. The relations observed between ambivalence and social support illustrate two possible facets in the experience of emotional ambivalence. Ambivalence involves the holding back of expression as well as expression coupled with excessive rumination. Individuals who are expressive yet conflicted may have developed skills to solicit support from others, yet feel guilty over their dependent behavior. In addition, the misrepresentation of emotion possible in the experience of ambivalence may also contribute to the mismatch of helping efforts by the observer and the actual need of the subject. Emotionally inhibited individuals, on the other hand, may wish to appear self-sufficient and are thus reluctant to express a desire for support. This would lead to the paradoxical prediction that the first type of ambivalent individual objectively receives social support, yet is subjectively dissatisfied with it. The second type of ambivalent individual, on the other hand, actually receives less social support yet expresses no displeasure. Observing how these individuals interact with others under conditions of distress may provide clues for understanding how support is elicited, or more likely, why it is not forthcoming from others.

Katz and Campbell (1994) demonstrated that emotionally ambivalent individuals showed less of a covariation between daily stressful events and negative affect. These authors attributed the asynchrony between event stress and mood to the emotional perseveration or rumination characteristic of ambivalent individuals.

King (1998) conducted three studies in which she examined the ability of emotionally conflicted individuals to correctly recognize the emotions of another. Ambivalent individuals reported more confusion in reading others' emotions, as measured through a self-report of emotional confusion in perceiving emotions as well as in videotaped emotional expressions. Her results dovetail nicely with those reported by Emmons and Colby (1995) and suggest that one reason why ambivalent individuals may have less than satisfactory relationships is because they lack the skills needed to gauge emotional reactions in others.

RESOLVING GOAL CONFLICTS

The restoration of well-being, both physical and psychological, requires that competition between goals be eliminated or at least reduced to a manageable level. Processes of conflict resolution are discussed in Emmons et al. (1993). They range from the avoidance of conflict by distraction to elimination of one or more of the conflicting goals. To regain more lasting control over psychological well-being, conflicts must ultimately be resolved. Since only recently has a critical mass of research been achieved on conflict, it should come as no surprise that little progress has been made on understanding mechanisms of integration. Kluckhohn and Murray (1953), among others, believe that the ability to resolve competing aims is central in personality processes. Tactics for resolving conflict include goal prioritization, integration, appeal to higher values and principles, and, if need be, the abandonment of irreconcilable goals. Temporary control over distressing affect caused by conflict may be achieved via one of these strategies or by distracting oneself from the conflict through various defenses or other disattentional mechanisms. For instance, one may choose to identify one's goals at a lower level of abstraction (Emmons, 1992; Vallacher & Wegner, 1985), as high-level thinking about conflictual material is likely to be stressful (Pennebaker, 1989). Given that certain personality styles predispose toward conflict and that conflict tends to be stable over time (Emmons, 1989), gaining control over chronic, debilitating conflict requires additional work.

Specific strategies are likely to be most effective for individuals facing specific decisional conflicts where the pros and cons of each alternative can be clearly articulated. Unfortunately, our conflicts are not always so tidy. Conflicts may be vaguely formulated, are often highly emotional, and are probably not subject to rational decision-making processes. Conflicts may be unconscious, and the person needs to become aware of and express the conflicting impulses before resolution can be considered. Clients do not normally come into therapy and announce, "I have an intrapsychic goal conflict." Typically, a developmental crisis (getting married, leaving home, graduating, retiring) may activate concerns, resulting in a clashing of wishes and fears. The Gestalt two-chair technique might prove helpful here (Greenberg & Safran, 1987). Visualization using metaphorical language (e.g., imagining oneself stuck between a rock and a hard place) might be useful for clarifying both sides of the conflict.

Fortunately, the process of maturation itself may bring about some integration of conflicting aspects of the person. Colby (1996) has explored the association between identity formation and goal conflict. She suggests that the process of identity development can bring previously disparate and conflicting goals into harmony. Preliminary support for this hypothesis was found in a sample of college undergraduates. Students in the moratorium phase of identity development reported more goal conflicts compared with students who were characterized by other identity statuses. This implies that a higher-order organizational structure such as identity can result in the effective management of lower-level goal conflicts.

One of the best illustrations of how maturation might facilitate conflict reduction in a person's life can be illustrated by considering a participant in one of my first studies on personal strivings. Among his personal strivings, "Chief" (a pseudonym) possessed the following explosive goals: to "Satisfy my girlfriend sexually," "Pick up attractive girls," "Make my girlfriend feel guilty when she talks to guys," "Make attractive women notice me," and "Avoid letting my girlfriend know I am in contact with other girls." He correctly evaluated the degree of incompatibility between these various aims at Time 1. He was able to lead this dual life by keeping his strivings efficiently compartmentalized: His girlfriend lived in a town 150 miles from where Chief was attending school. One year later, while still in college, two of his goals were to "Keep my girlfriend happy" and "Meet women at school." Apparently, he had toned down his earlier ambitions. Two years later, now graduated from college, his striving was to "Tell my fiancée I love you"; there was no hint of other women in his goal hierarchy. Finally, 2 years after that, and 5 years after the initial assessment, Chief's strivings were to "Work hard at my job," "Spend time with my family," "Keep my wife happy," and "Let others know my morality." A remarkable transformation had taken place—a life fragmented had been replaced with a life of integrity—full of meaning and unity. Chief had found that which made his life meaningful, valuable, and purposeful.

PART II

Spirituality, Goals, and Intelligence

CHAPTER FIVE

Spiritual Strivings as Ultimate Concerns

Faith, classically understood, is not a separate dimension of life, a compartmentalized specialty. Faith is an orientation of the total person, giving purpose and goal to one's hopes and strivings, thoughts and actions . . . as such, faith is an integral part of one's character or personality.
                                              —FOWLER (1981, pp. 14, 92)

The first part of this book has laid the foundation for what is to come. In the first four chapters, I have presented the basics of a motivational approach to personality centered on personal goals, and explored the value of such an approach for understanding subjective well-being. In Chapter 3, I reviewed the existing research on personal goals and well-being. The research was organized into three domains: goal content, goal orientation, and goal structure. In this chapter, which begins Part II of the book, I return to the topic of goal content and introduce the notion of a "psychology of ultimate concerns": an attempt to scientifically examine spirituality within motivation and personality.

Since I first began collecting lists of personal strivings over a dozen years ago, there have always been strivings that have not been categorizable given existing coding categories, most of which were patterned after the thematic motivation literature. Although the motivational triad of achievement, affiliation–intimacy, and power are well represented in strivings, they fail to capture what for many people are their most valued goals and concerns. In particular, strivings pertaining to the transcendent realm of experience, most notably those making reference to God or some conception of the Divine, appeared with some degree of regularity in striving lists. In fact, they appeared frequently enough that recently

I began to take them seriously and examine "striving for the sacred" in more detail. The Fowler quotation that opens this chapter eloquently expresses a position that I wish to strongly endorse in this chapter and in the remainder of this book: Faith is integral to personality. As such, it should affect every level of personality and touch every level of the person, including those aspects that are reflected in recurrent goal concerns. This chapter is devoted to an exploration of spirituality through personal goals. Is it possible to reliably identify spiritual and religious concerns in goal strivings? If so, can spiritual strivings help account for long-term individual differences in subjective well-being?

THE PREVALENCE AND SCOPE OF RELIGION

A core premise in this chapter is that spirituality is not an isolated, compartmentalized set of beliefs and practices; rather, it is an integral part of daily life. It is not confined to sacred occasions and to sacred locations. As such, spiritual concerns ought to find expression in what a person says he or she is typically trying to do. What is the basis for believing that people will report strivings that reflect a concern with spiritual matters? Religion is a basic category of human experience. Approximately 3.5 billion people around the world consider religion, in one form or another, to be an important influence in their daily lives (Paloutzian, 1996). National surveys consistently report that the vast majority of the American population are concerned with spiritual issues. According to national surveys, (Gallup & Castelli, 1989), 90% of Americans say they believe in God or a supreme being, two-thirds of those surveyed say that religion plays either an important or very important role in their lives, 40% attend worship services once a week, 71% made financial contributions to churches last year (vs. 32% to educational institutions and 24% to hospitals), and 71% of Americans believe in an afterlife. Interest in a variety of spiritualities ranging from the contemplative traditions to evangelical Christianity is on the increase in the United States. It is not an overstatement to say that spirituality permeates human lives. Pithily and forcefully stated, and despite postmodern claims to the contrary, "God will not go away" (d'Aquili & Newberg, 1998).

Given the prevalence of religion in society, it would be surprising, then, if spiritual and religious concerns did not find expression in one form or another through personal goals. Social forces shape individual lives and personalities. At first glance, it might seem odd to speak of religious or spiritual goals the way one talks about achievement goals or health goals or financial goals. After all, religions are belief systems, full of doctrine, practices, rituals, and symbols. Yet we speak quite openly of a "spiritual quest" of searching for the sacred. A spiritual search is the attempt to identify what is sacred and worthy of devotion. In form, there is nothing inherently different about religious and spiritual goals in comparison to any other type of goal. Religious and spiritual goals, like other goals, are internal mental representations of desired states that a person has identified as important and is committed to working toward. These states include outcomes, events, or processes.

There is a long history of using goal language metaphorically to depict spiritual growth. In devotional writings, spiritual growth and spiritual maturity are viewed as a process of goal attainment, with the ultimate goal being intimacy with the Divine. For instance, Gregory of Nyssa (Danielou & Musurillo, 1961) saw the spiritual life as a race wherein spiritual growth is a never-ending process of striving toward perfection. St. Teresa of Avila, in her classic *The Interior Castle*, saw progress in the spiritual life as a continuous striving toward greater depth and to the core of one's being, each step moving us closer to a vision of the ultimate. Similarly, the New Testament writer Paul, in his letter to the Philippians, wrote that "forgetting what is behind and straining toward that which is ahead, I press onward toward the goal to win the prize for which God has called me heavenward in Christ Jesus" (Phillipians 3:13–14, *The NIV Bible*, 1984, [*NIV*]). Jonathan Edwards (1746/1959), in his classic *A Treatise Concerning Religious Affections*, described "holy desire," which according to Edwards is reflected in a "longing, hungering, and thirsting after God" (p. 104). In content and function, however, there are substantial differences between spiritual goals and other types of goals, some of which will be explored in this chapter and in the next.

An examination of strivings that participants have spontaneously generated in past research does indeed seem to indicate spiritual concerns. For example, participants typically report strivings of trying to "Be aware of the spiritual meaningfulness of my life," "Discern and follow God's will for my life," "Bring my life in line with my beliefs," and "Communicate my faith with other people." Spirituality does appear to be a motivating force in people's lives. It seems likely that such motivational concerns would find expression in the goals that people report they are typically trying to seek in their everyday lives. One of the functions of a religious belief system and a religious worldview is that it provides "an ultimate vision of what people should be striving for in their lives" (Pargament & Park, 1995, p. 15) and the strategies to reach those ends. Similarly, Apter (1985) sees the religious state of mind as "telic," providing a guide to "the most serious and far-ranging goals there can possibly be" (p. 69). Values and goals occupy a prominent position in Richards and Bergin's (1997) hierarchical analysis of the concept of a metaphysical *weltanschauung*. One's worldview influences materialistic, relational, and spiritual and religious goals, which in turn determine life-styles and behaviors. The latter are the units of analysis most familiar to quality-of-life researchers, yet with respect to well-being, latent belief systems and resulting values and goals may be where the most significant action occurs.

DEFINING SPIRITUALITY THROUGH GOALS

It has become commonplace for authors to begin research articles and chapters on the psychology of religion with definitions of what exactly they mean by religion and spirituality. I will not depart from convention, and will also grapple with the definitional problem: How are spiritual/religious goals to be defined and assessed? Religion is an extraordinarily diverse, multifaceted construct (Batson, Schoenrade, & Ventis, 1992). Batson et al. (1992) depict religion as (1) unique—religious experience and religious concerns are more comprehensive and central to a person's life than are other concerns; (2) psychologically complex—religious experience involves a complex array of variables, including emotions, beliefs, attitudes, values, behaviors, and social environments; and (3) diverse—the experience and expression of religion of different individuals can be very different. Achieving conceptual clarity and methodological precision thus become challenges for the researcher intent on studying spiritual or religious units of analysis.

It is important to acknowledge that there is no agreed-upon definition of religion. It has been said that there is no more difficult word to define than "religion." In a conclusion that is cited more often than is any definition of religion, Yinger (1967) stated that "any definition of religion is likely to be satisfactory only to its author" (p. 18). This is primarily because religion is inward and subjective, highly individualized, and emotionally charged. Yet it is important to arrive at some consensus about the meaning of the term if progress is to be made in advancing research in the psychology of religion. While some authors have shied away from providing concrete definitions of the terms "spiritual" and "religious," there are no shortages of definitions. Some representative attempts at defining these richly complex terms are shown in Table 5.1.

Spirituality is typically defined quite broadly, with the term encompassing a search for meaning, for unity, for connectedness, for transcendence, for the highest of human potential. Religion and spirituality have generally been defined as that realm of life which is concerned with ultimate purpose and meaning in life, a set of principles and ethics to live by, commitment to God or a higher power, a recognition of the tran-

TABLE 5.1. Some Definitions of Religion and Spirituality

"*Religion* . . . the inner experience of the individual when he senses a Beyond, especially as evidenced by the effect of this experience on his behavior when he actively attempts to harmonize his life with the Beyond" (Clark, 1958, p. 22).

"*Spirituality* is a process by which individuals recognize the importance of orienting their lives to something nonmaterial that is beyond or larger than themselves . . . so that there is an acknowledgment of and at least some dependence upon a higher power, or Spirit" (Martin & Carlson, 1988, p. 59).

"At its core, *spirituality* consists of all the beliefs and activities by which individuals attempt to relate their lives to God or to a divine being or some other conception of a transcendent reality" (Wuthnow, 1998, p. vii).

"*Religion* is a system of symbols which acts to establish powerful, persuasive, and long-lasting moods and motivations by formulating conceptions of a general order of existence and clothing these conceptions with such an aura of factuality that the moods and motivations seem uniquely realistic" (Geertz, 1966, p. 90).

"*Spiritual* means believing in, valuing, or devoted to some higher power than what exists in the corporeal world . . . *religious* applies to any organized religion" (Worthington, Kurusu, McCullough, & Sandage, 1996, p. 449).

"*Spirituality* and *religion* are grounded in a dimension of reality beyond the boundaries of the strictly empirically perceived, material world. . . . The term *religion* has come to signify for many the codified, institutionalized, and ritualized expressions of peoples' communal connections to the Ultimate . . . *spirituality* is a deep sense of belonging, of wholeness, of connectedness, and of openness to the infinite" (Kelly, 1995, pp. 4–5).

"*Religion* is the sphere of human activity that includes (a) belief in a supernatural being or beings, and belief that human beings will establish a personal relationship with that being or beings, (b) certain rites and beliefs that are sanctioned by supernatural reality, (c) the division of life into the sacred and profane, (d) belief that the supernatural world communicates through human messengers, (e) the attempt to order life in harmony with supernatural designs, (f) belief that revealed truth supersedes other human efforts at understanding the world, and (g) the practice of creating a community of believers" (Beit-Hallahmi, 1989, pp. 11–12).

"*Religion* is concerned with a dimension that transcends mundane reality" (Wulff, 1997, p. 2).

scendent in everyday experience, a selfless focus, and a set of beliefs and practices that is designed to facilitate a relationship with the transcendent. This definition is consistent with a number of authors who, while acknowledging the diversity of meaning, affirm as a common core meaning of spirituality/religion that of the recognition of a transcendent, meta-empirical dimension of reality (e.g., Kelly, 1995; Pargament & Park, 1995; Worthington, Kurusu, McCullough, & Sandage, 1996). For example, Martin and Carlson (1988) define spirituality as "a process by which individuals recognize the importance of orienting their lives to something nonmaterial that is beyond or larger than themselves . . . so that there is an acknowledgment of and at least some dependence upon a higher power, or Spirit" (p. 59).

Religion is a broader concept than spirituality, since religion may involve more than a search for the sacred. Religion may, for example, be a route toward intimacy, meaning, status, comfort, or a variety of other end-states (Pargament, 1997). Although I will use the term "spiritual strivings" throughout this chapter, spiritual strivings contain both conventional religious themes as well as more personalized expressions of spiritual concern. Although my concern in this chapter is primarily with "religious spirituality," it is certainly the case that other, nonreligious, humanistic versions of the concept imbue human strivings as well. The challenge will be to capture both forms of "higher strivings" in an objective, reliable, and scientific manner. As in any psychological accounting of spiritual processes or religious processes, this discussion makes no assumptions regarding the existence of spiritual realities or the truth claims of any particular religious system.

ULTIMATE CONCERN AND ULTIMATE CONCERNS

Central to both religion and spirituality is a search process (Pargament, 1997). Searches imply that there is something to be found; those end-states are goals. A spiritual search involves the attempt to identify what is sacred and worthy of being committed to. The sacred refers to God, or related names for God, such as divine power, Supreme Being, Ultimate Reality, or Ultimate Truth. Recall that personal strivings represent recurring and relatively enduring concerns, in that they pertain to states of mind that persist over time and across situations. This is in contrast to "current concerns" (Klinger, 1977), defined as the interim between commitment to a goal and its successful attainment or disengagement. Religious or spiritual strivings may be different from nonreligious (secular) strivings as religious experience may be different from other types of psychological experience. Spiritual strivings can be conceptualized as "ultimate concerns," following Tillich (1957), as discussed in Chapter 1. Religion is a person's ultimate concern. Ultimate concern was described in Chapter 1 as that in which maximal value is invested, which possesses the power to center one's life, and which demands "total surrender" (Tillich, 1957, p. 3). Spiritual personal strivings reflect an acknowledgment of the Ultimate or Absolute and either a collective (religious) or individualistic (spiritual) desire to orient one's life to the Ultimate. In a similar vein, Hebrew scholar and Rabbi Abraham Heschel (1955) depicted the search for God as "the search for ultimacy" (p. 125). The ultimate is that beyond which nothing else exists or is possible. Spiritual strivings, then, become the way in which ultimate concern is encountered in people's lives. From this perspective, strivings are either preliminary or ultimate; ultimate strivings are those that are centered on a search for the sacred. The word ultimate comes from the Latin *ultimus*, meaning last or most distant. According to *Webster's Encyclopedic Unabridged Dictionary,* the ultimate is the highest, best, greatest, or most extreme of its kind; it is not subsidiary to others. Ultimate concern, then, is that above which no other concerns exist—it is literally at the end of the striving line.

Contemporary writers have gone to great pains to differentiate spirituality from religion, and psychologists who bristle at the label of religiousness generally have no quarrel with defining themselves as spiritual (Shafranske, 1996). One common thread that appears to transcend the diverse meanings of spirituality and religion is the notion of *ultimacy.* Clark (1958) found that in a survey of members of the Society for the Scientific Study of Religion the most frequent response given to the question of what is religion involved supernatural concepts related to the ultimate. Allport (1950) defined a mature religious sentiment as "a disposition to respond favorably . . . to objects or principles that the individual regards as of *ultimate importance* in his own life, and as having to do with what he regards as permanent or central in the nature of things" (p. 56). Spirituality has been defined as that which "involves ultimate and personal truths" (Wong 1998, p. 364). Elkins (1988) defines spirituality as "a way of being and experiencing that which comes about through awareness of a transcendent dimension and that is characterized by certain identifiable values in regard to self, others, nature, life and whatever one considers to be the Ultimate" (p. 10). Spirituality has been said to refer to how an individual "lives meaningfully with ultimacy, his or her response to the deepest truths of the universe as he or she apprehends these" (Bregman & Thierman, 1995, p. 149).

Given the preceding definition and characteristics of "the ultimate," is there a contradiction between using the language of ultimate concern to refer to strivings that reflect everyday goals and concerns? In other words, can there be an ultimacy of the vernacular? I am assuming that ultimate concern, that is, a concern with identifying the sacred and orienting one's life around it, will be manifested in recurring and enduring concerns that I am calling strivings. No single striving is, of course, likely to do justice to the rich formulations of Tillich and other theologically mindful writers who have discussed religion as ultimate concern. But spiritual strivings are likely to be significant for the person who holds them. The discussion by Pargament (1997) is ed-

ifying in this respect. He defines spirituality as "the search for significance in ways related to the sacred" (p. 32). As we will see in later
chapters, however, sacredness appears in many shapes and forms,
from the most magnificent aims to the seemingly most mundane pursuits. Almost any striving can become sacralized through a process of
sanctification, a setting aside of the striving for a holy purpose. I will
return to the theme of sanctified striving later in this chapter. It is sufficient to say here that even the ultimate can appear in daily goals in
matters that may appear, at least on the surface, to be insignificant or
quite ordinary (see Pargament, 1997, Chap. 2, for a sophisticated discussion of this point).

The Uniqueness of Ultimate Concerns

One of the primary suppositions of this book is that ultimate concerns
are unique aspects of personality, functioning in some senses in similar
ways to other goals, while at the same time being of a different nature
than other types of strivings that are more familiar to personality researchers. Batson et al. (1992) suggest that religious concerns are unique
in that they are more comprehensive in scope and are more central to
who a person is than are everyday concerns. Ultimate concerns strike at
the heart of who a person is; they are all-consuming and self-defining.
This quote from Ian Barbour (1960), a professor of physics and religion,
elegantly describes the link between religion and ultimacy: "Religious
faith refers to a man's ultimate trust, his most basic commitments, what
he bets his life on, the final basis by which he justifies all his other values. The religious question is precisely about the object of a person's devotion; it asks to what or to whom a person gives his ultimate
allegiance" (p. 210).

A more colorful depiction of the psychology of ultimate concerns
was voiced by personologist Henry Murray (1960): "A man's ultimate
concern is whether he spends an eternity of years in the best place imaginable or in the worst place imaginable. Seventy multipleasured years on
earth are of little worth when weighed against an endless age of sizzling
in the underground; and a lifetime of vexation, misery, and woe are tol-
erable if after the fever of life one is destined to enjoy a trillion years of
bliss" (p. 148).

Virtually all of the writing on ultimate concerns, be it from theologians, scientists, or philosophers, leads to the empirically testable hypothesis that ultimate concerns should assume a level of primacy
within a person's overall goal hierarchy. Empirical research bearing on
this hypothesis will be presented later in this chapter and in the next
chapter.

Previous Research Attempts to Identify Spiritual Goals

A review of the goal literature yielded only a couple of efforts to include spiritual or religious concerns in goal-content categories. In their taxonomy of human goals, Ford and Nichols (1987) include the superordinate theme of "subjective organization goals," under which appear unity goals and goals for transcendence. Unity goals are goals that involve "experiencing a profound or spiritual sense of connectedness, harmony, or oneness with people, nature, or a greater power; avoiding feelings of disunity or disorganization" (p. 295). Transcendent goals are those that involve "experiencing optimal or extraordinary states of functioning; avoiding feeling trapped within the boundaries of ordinary experience" (Ford, 1994, p. 200). Unfortunately, no evidence for the validity of these categories is presented.

Lapierre, Bouffard, and Bastin (1997) categorized the personal aspirations of a sample of several hundred elderly persons in Canada. Using a methodology similar to the strivings assessment method, participants were asked to complete 23 sentence stems beginning with phrases such as "I would like. . . . " and "I wish. . . . " Transcendental concerns represented one of 10 major motivational categories that emerged from a content analysis of goals. Two types of goals made up this category— religious ("to go to church," "to go to heaven") and eschatological ("to have a good death"). The method used by Lapierre et al. is notable in that participants were able to freely express their conscious goals and wishes in their own words, thus capitalizing on the strength of open-ended goal assessment methods. This is a procedure that may have wider applicability in the assessment of spirituality and religiousness.

Advantages of a Goal-Based Approach to Spirituality

Personal strivings offer an advantageous approach for both conceptualizing and measuring spirituality. In addition, spirituality can enlarge our conception of human motivational strivings to include the realm of the sacred. Religious attitudes and behaviors are most often the variables of choice in empirical research on religiousness and subjective well-being. Many of these are single-item measures of questionable reliability and validity. National surveys have regularly reported that approximately 64% of the American population are members of a church or synagogue, while about 40% attend worship services on a weekly basis (Koenig, 1997). The majority of research on religious and spiritual factors on health has relied nearly exclusively on this church-based population. While substantial advances have been made in understanding religion's influence on health, the overreliance of churched populations as research participants limits the generalizability of the role of spiritual factors in people's lives. The spirituality of the remaining unchurched population has not been studied systematically. How does spirituality operate in the daily lives of individuals who are not associated with a traditional religious faith? Conventional measures such as worship attendance may be inappropriate for persons who hold no particular institutional affiliation. A goal-based measure of spirituality offers a perspective that transcends measures of denominational affiliation, retrospective reports of church attendance or prayer or other spiritual activity, and general attitudes toward religion to encompass the diversity of daily goals, enduring strivings, and ultimate concerns of a spiritually oriented lifestyle under the same theoretical umbrella or "sacred canopy" (Berger, 1967). The personal strivings approach also exploits the power of a combined nomothetic–idiographic assessment strategy. It reflects the idiosyncratic ways in which individuals strive to obtain or maintain a concern with the sacred in their everyday lives. At the same time, it allows for conclusions to be drawn about the relation between spiritual goals and well-being that generalize across persons, independent of the unique expression of spiritual concern within that person.

    To illustrate briefly what a personal goals perspective can offer the scientific study of spirituality, consider two hypothetical individuals, A. W. and J. I. On conventional measures of religiousness, such as worship attendance, prayer frequency, and importance of religion they appear very similar to each other. In fact, they might achieve identical scores on these indices. Yet these surface similarities obscure fundamental differences in structural and functional properties of their spiritual goal hierarchies. A.W. has the goals to "Get closer to God," to "Cultivate spiritual meaning in my life," and to "Discern God's will for my life." Furthermore, he appraises these goals as extremely important, but has a rather vague notion of how he will actually go about pursuing them, and sees them as conflicting with more mundane pursuits in the realms of work and family. J. I., on the other hand, has included among his strivings to "Memorize five Scripture verses a day," "Be forgiving when dealing with my ex-spouse," and "Witness to others when opportunities arise." J. I.'s relatively more focused and concrete strivings, for which he perceives a high likelihood of attainment, are likely to have measurably different effects on his physical and mental health compared to A.W.'s negative appraisals of his more abstract goals. The research on level of abstraction as a goal orientation and well-being described in Chapter 3 demonstrated that a trade-off between manageability and meaningfulness of goals is most conducive to psychological and physical well-being.

PREVIOUS RESEARCH ON SPIRITUALITY
AND PSYCHOLOGICAL WELL-BEING

The research literature on mental health and religiousness is voluminous and, while previously rather chaotic, substantial recent progress has been made. Several comprehensive reviews have recently been published (Batson et al., 1992; Brown, 1994; Gartner, 1996; Koenig, 1998; Levin & Tobin, 1995; Schumaker, 1992; Ventis, 1995). Religious commitment and participation consistently emerge as significant contributors of quality-of-life indications such as life satisfaction, happiness, and meaning in life (Chamberlain & Zika, 1992; Diener, 1984; Levin & Tobin, 1995; Poloma & Pendleton, 1990). Poloma and Pendleton (1990) provided a comprehensive critique of the research literature on religiosity and domains of general well-being. Employing eight measures of religiosity, these authors found that religiosity was an important predictor of general life satisfaction, existential well-being, and overall happiness. Ventis (1995) reviewed over 100 studies and reported a mixture of results: some studies find positive effects of religiousness on well-being, some find negative effects, and some find no effects at all. The general conclusion that can be drawn from this literature is that it makes little sense to ask whether religiousness is related to mental health. Asking this type of question would be akin to asking whether attachment style is related to well-being. In either case, the answer is a resounding "it depends." It depends on how both spiritual–religious and mental health variables are defined and measured. At a minimum, critical distinctions need to be made between extrinsic (religion as a means to an end) and intrinsic (religion as a way of life) religiousness, with measures of the former generally showing negative correlations with well-being and measures of the latter positive correlations with well-being (Ventis, 1995). Some have argued (Kirkpatrick & Hood, 1990; Pargament, 1992) that even a rudimentary distinction between intrinsic and extrinsic religiousness fails to begin to capture the complexity inherent in the construct of religiosity or spirituality. Ryan, Rigby, and King (1993) proposed that *religious internalization*, or the degree to which religious beliefs and values are self-determined as opposed to coerced, is a critical factor influencing mental health.

In terms of psychological or subjective well-being, distinctions need to be made between the presence of positive well-being (e.g., happiness, morale, life satisfaction) and the absence of negative states such as depression, anxiety, and physical symptoms (as I noted in Chapter 2). Distinctions should also be made between affective well-being, such as happiness, and cognitive well-being, such as life satisfaction and meaning in life. Depending on how each set of variables is measured, one can find evidence for either the helpful or harmful effects of religiousness on mental health. Yet as Batson and Burris (1994) persuasively argue, research needs to move beyond the rhetoric of "celebrating or castigating religion based on extreme examples" (p. 150). The way to do this is by conducting research that acknowledges the complexity of each construct and attempts to be true to this complexity by striving for systematic measurement of the variables involved.

Spiritual Strivings and Well-Being

Emmons, Cheung, and Tehrani (1998) investigated the relation between spiritual strivings, emotional well-being, and overall life satisfaction. We employed several different outcome measures of well-being and sampled both college-age and older adults in the local community. Participants in three samples generated lists of their personal strivings, which were then coded for spirituality. All participants completed a variety of psychological well-being measures, chosen to represent an array of well-being variables. Some of these were multiple measures over time using a daily report methodology, whereas others were single-session questionnaire measures. To augment the self-reports, spouse reports of well-being were obtained for in the community samples.

The study was designed to address the following questions:

1. Can spirituality be reliably assessed through personal goal strivings?
2. If so, do spiritual strivings contribute unique amounts of variance in the prediction of well-being?
3. If spiritual strivings are related to well-being, what are some of the cognitive-motivational mechanisms by which they do? In other words, are spiritual strivings appraised differently than nonspiritual strivings?
4. Are there gender differences in the relation between spiritual strivings and well-being?
5. Does the relation between spiritual strivings and well-being depend upon the particular well-being outcome that is used?

In general, we expected that the proportion of spiritual strivings in a person's total goal system, a rough index of spiritual concern, would be positively associated with measures of psychological well-being. Strivings represent intrinsic goals that a person desires to accomplish, and it has been previously established that intrinsic measures of religiousness tend to predict higher levels of well-being. One may engage in strivings for extrinsic reasons, but, as Sheldon and Kasser (1995) found, most personal strivings tend to be rated high in self-determination.

Coding Strivings for Spirituality

Beginning with the definition of spirituality established earlier, my students and I set out to systematically examine spiritual content in personal strivings. Proceeding as we had for other striving thematic categories, we sought to develop a set of coding criteria that could reliably classify strivings as spiritual based on a categorical accounting of the target of the individual striving as directed toward the sacred. The main purpose of the study was to develop and test the validity of this coding system in the prediction of psychological well-being in various samples.

In developing criteria for identifying spiritual content in personal strivings, there were two primary considerations. First, the criteria had to adequately represent the multidimensionality of religiousness. A second concern was that the criteria be general enough to capture spiritual concern in as noncontroversial, nonsectarian, and inclusive a manner as possible, without being so general as to be useless. Although spirituality is often associated with religious beliefs and practices, we did not wish to rule out nonconventional religiousness. Beginning with James's (1902) distinction between feelings, acts, and experiences, psychologists have historically partitioned religious experience into meaningful clusters of activity. Glock (1962; Glock & Stark, 1965) developed a multidimensional representation of religiosity that lends itself to a coding of spiritual strivings by dividing religiosity into knowledge, feelings, practice, belief, and effects. Of these, knowledge, feelings, and practice are most likely to capture the manifestation of spirituality in strivings. We initially utilized this classification system for the coding of strivings. Thus, spiritual strivings are those that reflected (1) increasing one's knowledge of a higher power ("Increase my knowledge of the Bible," "Seek God's will in my life," "Learn about God's creation in the world"); (2) developing or maintaining a relationship with a higher power ("Deepen my relationship with God," "Learn to tune into a higher power throughout the day," "Increase my faith in God"); (3) attempting to live or exercise one's spiritual beliefs in daily life ("Not be judgmental," "Witness to others," "Treat others with compassion"). These criteria, based primarily on previous psychological theory and research on religion, were developed in Phase 1.

An examination of theological writings on spirituality and spiritual formation led to the inclusion of additional criteria in Phase 2. The core component of spirituality is reflected in the notion of "transcendence." The influential theologian Reinhold Niebuhr (1941) affirmed that transcendence is the striving toward some possibility not present in the material world (Finger, 1997). Strivings that are oriented above and beyond the self, that reflect an integration of the individual with larger and more complex units, or that reflect deepening or maintaining a relationship with a higher power reflect a desire to transcend the self. Strivings are coded as spiritual if they reflect concern for an integration of the person with larger and more complex units: with humanity, nature, the cosmos (to "Achieve union with the totality of existence," "Immerse myself in nature and be part of it," "Approach life with mystery and awe"). Strivings are content analyzed by trained coders for the presence of self-transcendent themes. Coding strivings in this manner allows for greater inclusivity than do many existing measures of spirituality or religiousness and will likely be sensitive to the diversity of spiritual expression in a religiously pluralistic culture. At this point in time the criteria remain open; it is anticipated that the existing criteria will be refined and additional ones will be developed based upon the outcomes of this research and continued examination of relevant literatures. Examples of spiritual strivings are shown in Table 5.2.

To supplement the self-reports, spouse reports of strivings were also obtained. Spouses were asked to provide a list of strivings that they believed characterized their partner. In response to "What do you think your partner typically tries to do?" they were provided with two blank lines in which to complete the stem "He/she typically tries to. . . . " They were instructed not to confer with their partners and not to discuss the study until the questionnaire packets had been mailed back to us. An additional measure of religious goals was employed with the college sam-

TABLE 5.2. Examples of Spiritual Strivings

"Share my faith with the receptive in a gentle, loving way."
"Not weigh material things as being more important than spiritual things."
"Praise God everyday whether my situation is good or bad."
"Move further along the path of knowing and loving God."
"Improve myself daily—whether it be mentally, spiritually, or physically."
"Spend time reading the Bible every morning."
"Volunteer my time and talent in my church."
"Say my prayers daily and deepen my understanding of the Bahai teachings."
"Be a forgiving person."
"Be more Christlike in character."
"Remain true to God while trying to please my nonbelieving spouse."
"Take a Sabbath."
"Find and discover truths about life—develop a philosophy for meaning."
"Fulfill my religious obligations."
"Strive to have a closer relationship to God."

ple in order to augment the spiritual striving measure. Participants were presented with a list of 10 religious goals and were asked to rate the importance of each goal in their current lives. This group of goals, taken from clustering analysis of a goal taxonomy questionnaire (Chulef, Read, & Walsh, 1996), consisted of the following: achieving salvation; being honest; being charitable; finding higher meaning in life, harmony, or oneness; helping others; pleasing God; engaging in religious traditions; maintaining religious faith; having wisdom; and having firm values. Participants rated the importance of these 10 goals on a 5-point scale.

Major Results

In the three samples, the proportion of spiritual strivings ranged from an average of 8% in the college sample to an average of 28% in the two community samples. Interestingly, in none of the samples were significant differences found in the proportion of spiritual strivings endorsed by men and women. Nearly all research on religiousness has found that women score higher on conventional measures of religiousness. Clearly, some of the reasons for gender equivalence in strivings deserves further study. The proportion of spiritual strivings within the person's overall striving profile was significantly associated with rated importance of religion, attendance at religious services, the frequency of prayer, and a measure of intrinsic religiousness (Gorsuch & McPherson, 1989). The checklist of religious goals was moderately correlated with the proportion of spiritual strivings, providing additional validity for the strivings measure. With respect to subjective well-being, spiritual strivings tended to be related to higher levels of well-being, especially to greater purpose in life and to both marital and overall life satisfaction. Spiritual strivings appear to make a unique contribution to well-being even when potentially overlapping item content is taken into account. Correlations between spiritual strivings and well-being indicators for the community sample are shown in Table 5.3.

Spiritual strivings accounted for significant variance in well-being outcomes beyond the religious variables of attendance, rated importance, and prayer frequency. The associations between spiritual goals and well-being were generally stronger for women than for men, and held when using spouse reports of strivings as well as spouse reports of well-being. Spiritual strivings were rated as more important and as requiring more effort, and were engaged in for more intrinsic reasons than were nonspiritual strivings. Spiritual strivings were also associated with lower levels of goal conflict. Results indicated that it is possible to reliably assess spiritual motivation in personal goals, and that individual

TABLE 5.3. Correlations between Spiritual Strivings and Well-Being

Well-being measure	Combined (N = 100)	Females (N = 50)	Males (N = 50)	Spir. Int (N = 100)
% Happy	.26**	.36**	.12	.16
% Unhappy	−.33**	−.42**	−.25	−.33**
SWLS	.48**	.58**	.36*	.43**
CESD	−.29**	−.38**	−.21	−.24*
Neuroticism	−.30**	−.46**	−.17	−.25**
DAS	.36**	.41**	.32*	.30**

Note. Spir. Int, proportion of spiritual strivings, controlling for proportion of intimacy strivings; SWLS, Satisfaction With Life Scale; CESD, Center for Epidemiological Studies Depression Scale; DAS, Dyadic Adjustment Scale.
*p < .05; **p < .01.

differences in spiritual motivation are related to various components of well-being. Moreover, the correlations between the proportion of spiritual strivings and well-being measures were stronger than any other type of striving that has been studied, exceeding those for intimacy, power, or generativity. It does appear to be the case that, when it comes to well-being, "all goals are not created equal" (Ryan et al., 1996, p. 7). As a basic category of human experience, spirituality is revealed through ultimate concerns that center on the sacred. When people orient their lives around the attainment of spiritual ends, they tend to experience their lives as worthwhile, unified, and meaningful.

When Spiritual Striving Fails

While spiritual strivings tend to be associated with higher levels of well-being, it should not be assumed that spirituality guarantees emotional bliss. Religion is not necessarily the royal road to happiness. High-level religious strivings, if not accompanied by concrete plans and strategies for attainment, might be experienced as a source of frustration. Like other high-level strivings, successful self-regulation hinges on the identification of progress indicators. Unlike other high-level strivings, though, spiritual strivings might provide sufficient meaning and purpose to offset the uneasiness associated with other forms of abstract strivings. Serious religious mindfulness can make a person increasingly uneasy about his or her shortcomings, particularly when he or she is strongly committed to a goal of living a virtuous life. Although religions are often accused of burdening a person with guilt, dissatisfaction can be desirable if it is used as fuel for constructive life change. People might also become legalistic about their lower level, concrete spiritual strivings, rigidly holding to goals and means in an obsessive–compulsive fashion (Vergote, 1988).

The legalist, according to Bixler (1988), "wishes to legislate every area of life and thus tends to concentrate on behavioral and religious minutiae" (p. 335). Low-level spiritual strivings might be indicative of legalistic tendencies, particularly when combined with inflexible strategies for their attainment or the inability to link them with higher-order meaningful goals.

Appraisals of Spiritual Strivings

Although significant associations between spiritual content in goals and indicators of subjective well-being were established in the Emmons, Cheung, and Tehrani (1998) study, the mechanisms responsible for these links remain largely unknown. One of the advantages of a mixed nomothetic–idiographic strategy is that it permits quantitative indices to be derived from qualitative information from individual persons. Perhaps spiritual and nonspiritual strivings differ in appraisals across specific appraisal dimensions. If spiritual strivings are appraised relatively more favorably along motivational dimensions of expectancy, purpose, effort, and the like, this would be suggestive of the processes through which spiritual strivings enable positive mental health outcomes. More generally, such an analysis would extend the religion–mental health link by exploring motivational mechanisms by which personal religiousness might affect mental and physical health outcomes (Koenig, 1997; Schumaker, 1992). We did find that spiritual strivings were significantly more valued, perceived as less effortful and difficult, more attainable, more likely to be engaged in for intrinsic reasons, and as more instrumental for accomplishing other strivings than nonspiritual strivings. In Table 5.4, it can be seen that participants appraised their spiritual strivings less ambivalently and as more important, and rated success as more probable than for nonspiritual strivings.

All in all, spiritual strivings were appraised more favorably than were nonspiritual strivings, thus suggesting a means by which spiritual strivings can impact well-being. As reviewed in Chapter 3, goal-specific appraisals have been shown to be significant predictors of subjective well-being. The specific pattern of appraisals that characterize spiritual strivings (greater value, instrumentality and intrinsicness, and less conflict, effort, and difficulty) has been associated with a variety of well-being indicators (Emmons, 1996; Palys & Little, 1983; Ryan et al., 1996).

Implications of the Emmons, Cheung, and Tehrani (1998) Study

A personal strivings approach to measuring spirituality was designed to be able to reliably identify religious and spiritual content in personal

TABLE 5.4. Correlations between Striving Assessment Scales and
Spiritual Strivings

SAS	Combined (N = 100)	Females (N = 50)	Males (N = 50)
Importance	.20*	.16	.24*
Ambivalence	−.22*	−.21	−.26*
Probability of success	.40**	.45**	.33*
Difficulty	−.26*	−.23*	−.31*

Note. SAS, Striving Assessment Scales.
*p < .05; **p < .01.

goals, and to be sensitive to individual differences in the meaning and
expression of spirituality in everyday life. Taken as a whole, the research
of Emmons, Cheung, and Tehrani (1998) supports the claim that striving for spiritual ends in life promotes long-term subjective well-being. It
also makes marriage better. Spiritual strivings were generally related to
higher levels of individual well-being as well as to increased marital satisfaction, and this relationship generally held across the measures of
well-being in the community samples. Moreover, these relations held
when controlling for intimacy strivings, one of the few striving content
categories that has been shown to relate to well-being in previous research (Emmons, 1991). Theoretically, one would expect overlap between spirituality and intimacy, given the core component of relational
connectedness inherent in each construct. As researchers in the mental
health and physical health fields have been reporting, there is a spiritual
reality to people's lives that can be reliably and objectively assessed, and
that has measurable consequences for both individual and relational
well-being.

The relation between spiritual strivings and well-being was not limited to the self-report realm. The strivings attributed by marital partners
to each other successfully predicted each person's level of well-being separately. This is the first reported study that has capitalized on the ability
of knowledgeable others to report personal strivings, and to link these
observer reports to well-being outcomes. Evidently spirituality manifests
itself in concerns that are readily observable to significant others, and
there also appears to be considerable agreement between spouse-
attributed and self-attributed spirituality in strivings.

The relations between spiritual strivings and well-being in the
Emmons, Cheung, and Tehrani (1998) study were correlational in nature. I assume, as has previous research on religiousness and well-being,
that spiritual variables (in this case, goals) are causally prior to well-

being and thus contribute to well-being, rather than the converse. The scant empirical research on religious conversion speaks more to the issue of causality, and studies that have assessed well-being before and after conversion tend to report a postconversion increase in well-being (Blaine & Crocker, 1995). Strivings also appear to be relatively stable over time, both in terms of content and appraisal ratings (Emmons, 1989), increasing the likelihood that well-being is a function of what the person is trying to do, rather than vice versa. Clearly, though, much additional research is needed to refine the present findings and to determine if the patterns observed here replicate and extend prospectively over time.

Striving for Significance and the Sanctification of Personal Goals

Everyday spirituality, the kind that is measured through personal strivings, appears to promote psychological well-being. It has been suggested that much of the power of a spiritual or religious lifestyle comes from the human ability to sanctify secular objects (Pargament, 1997). To sanctify means to make holy. Holiness is a formal characteristic of particular objects, persons, and places. To sanctify is to set apart from the ordinary or mundane and to dedicate to a particular purpose or use. According to the scriptures, certain vessels from the potter's shop were set aside for use by the priests officiating in the temple and became "holy vessels" (Romans 9:21, *NIV*). Another meaning of the term pertains to the process by which persons are made pure or holy. It thus refers to moral goodness or spiritual worth (Erickson, 1985). According to Christian theology, this form of sanctification is a supernatural work; it is something done by God, not something people do to themselves (Erickson, 1985).

Personal strivings in life can become sanctified or imbued with a sense of the holy. As a consequence, they are likely to be appraised differently than are secularized strivings. When work is seen as a calling rather than a job, or as an opportunity to serve God, work-related strivings take on new significance (Davidson & Caddell, 1994; Novak, 1996), In the same vein, when parenting is viewed as a sacred responsibility (Dollahite, 1998), it is likely to be approached differently than when viewed in purely secular terms. Even as seemingly an ordinary activity as running can become imbued with spiritual significance. In the extraordinary film *Chariots of Fire*, Eric Liddell reflects on the deeper significance of running in revealing that "when I run, I feel His pleasure." Religion influences the way in which people think about themselves, their families, their jobs, and their goals. To quote Pargament (1997), "the search for meaning, community, self, a better world are

likely to be transformed when they are invested with a sacred character"
(p. 12). Mahoney et al. (in press) and Pargament (1997) found that
when marital partners viewed their relationship as imbued with divine
qualities, they reported greater levels of marital satisfaction, more constructive problem-solving behaviors, decreased marital conflict, and
greater commitment to the relationship, compared to couples who saw
their marriage in a less sacred light.

Mechanisms Linking Spiritual Goals with Well-Being

What advantage for psychological well-being is there in holding spiritual
goals? What theoretical mechanism might explain why those who commit themselves to spiritual goals live a life that is more meaningful and
rewarding? To answer this question, one needs to consider what is most
essential to spiritual strivings. They may have an empowering function;
individuals are more likely to persevere in these strivings, even under difficult circumstances. People admit that in today's culture their spiritual
strivings are not always socially sanctioned, yet they derive tremendous
meaning and purpose from them. Spiritual strivings are likely to provide
stability and support in times of crisis by reorienting people to what is
ultimately important in life. Perhaps the most important function of
spirituality, one that I will defend in the next chapter, is that it potentially can confer coherence upon the personality. Religion or spirituality
can provide a unifying philosophy of life and serve as an integrating and
stabilizing force in the face of constant environmental and cultural pressures that push for fragmentation (Allport, 1950; Tillich, 1957). Conflict or fragmentation is a source of stress that exerts a deleterious effect
on well-being (Chapter 4); thus psychic structures that facilitate the integration of personality elements should be associated with positive well-
being. I believe that this "coherence hypothesis" is a promising one, and
it is explored more fully in the next chapter.

Limitations of Spirituality through Strivings

Some limitations of measuring ultimate concern from personal strivings
should be mentioned. Although the personal strivings approach appears
to represent a heuristically useful way of conceptualizing personal spirituality, we must not assume that it reflects the sum total of a person's
spiritual life. Undoubtedly, there are significant aspects of personal spirituality that may not be manifested in and articulated through what the
person is "typically trying to do." For example, ideological beliefs regarding particular religious worldviews may or may not be revealed in
personal strivings. Nor necessarily would beliefs pertaining to life after

death, salvation and redemption, or other ultimate concerns automatically appear on someone's list of strivings. Rather, as a mixture of ideologically driven and experientially based goals, the strivings approach is likely to capture "pragmatic spirituality" and the translation of a broader spiritual orientation into daily commitments and concerns. It is important to note the boundary conditions of the strivings construct in deciding the contribution to the literature on personality, well-being, and spirituality that the striving approach makes.

With the emphasis on *personal* striving, is there a danger of losing the sacred core of spirituality? Or the communal core of traditional religious worship? These types of concerns caused me some uneasiness when I first applied the personal strivings framework to the study of spiritual and religious issues. There is risk that spiritual striving can become an expression of egoistic impulses, rather than a search for the divine. Strivings themselves can become idolatrous in that the object of concern is not truly the ultimate. Strivings for self-glorification can be dressed up in religious terminology, but that does not change the fact that the ultimate concern is with exaltation of the self. As Shore (1997) recently noted, spiritual growth can become defined in terms of personal goals—an exercise in personal subjectivity. But authentic spiritual growth involves replacing the self as the source of ultimate concern with family, community, humanity, and divinity (Shore, 1997). It involves the emptying of oneself. Unfortunately, there is no way of knowing for certain where one's ultimate focus is. It is possible to examine references to God (as one conceives of God) in striving lists as a criterion for spirituality through strivings. But how can one be certain that the subject is just engaging in God-talk devoid of authentic spirituality? An alternative is to look to the fruits of a spiritually oriented lifestyle. Tillich (1951) spoke of "existential disappointment," which he saw as the result of giving ultimate concern to that which is merely transitory and temporal. A life that is centered around authentic spiritual goal strivings ought to result in a life that is meaningful, valuable, and purposeful, and that is what the data on personal strivings appear to show.

Why Spirituality through Strivings?

Personal strivings would appear to hold promise as conceptual units for measuring personal spirituality. From the perspective of progress in the scientific study of spirituality, there may be significant advantages in a goal approach to spiritual and religious phenomena. Adopting a descriptive and explanatory framework that has proven useful in established areas of psychology (not to mention in living systems more generally) can lead to substantial advances in understanding spiritual processes and

how these relate to other aspects of the person. As Klinger (1998) so eloquently stated, "By bringing the more rarefied human pleasures into the
same framework as other goals, they can be construed as part of the
common affective currency of an individual's motivational economy"
(p. 35).

There are also personal advantages to considering one's spiritual
growth using the economy of strivings. Because it deals with the inner
life of the person, the strivings approach is ideal for examining spiritual
interiority and the process of spiritual formation across the life span.
Strivings provide both a window into naturally occurring personal spirituality as well as a potential intervention tool for cultivating the human
spirit. A goal-based approach conceives of spirituality as a dynamic process that has the potential to change in intensity and expression over
time and across situations. This necessitates assessment instruments that
can capture contextualized and highly idiosyncratic manifestations of
spiritual commitment that may be linked with specific developmental periods in life. In other words, spirituality may be expressed differently by
a person in his or her 20s than by someone in his or her 80s. Because it is
sensitive to temporal context, and because it deals with the inner life of
the person, the strivings approach is ideal for examining the process of
spiritual formation across the lifespan, as well as across different religious traditions. In Islam, for example, one might be a lifelong devoted
Muslim. In adulthood, one might take up Sufism (the mystical branch of
Islam), and, as a result, experience *fana* (self-annihilation in Allah). Earlier I suggested that strivings may arise from a conversion to a spiritual
or religious system, but striving for mystical realization can also occur in
one who is already deeply religious. By focusing inner awareness, the
strivings protocol offers a potent combination as a tool for spiritual
growth. The personal strivings method provides both a window into
naturally occurring personal spirituality as well as a potential intervention tool for cultivating the human spirit.

Future work might find it profitable to obtain separate indices of
experiential, cognitive, and behavioral aspects of spirituality and to distinguish between the goals of deepening spirituality and increasing or
maintaining religious involvement (Atchley, 1995). It may also be desirable, at some future point, to make further distinctions in different types
of spiritual striving, such as between high- and low-level spiritual goals,
given the differential pattern of correlates with well-being that I described in Chapter 3. Not all expressions of spiritual striving are likely to
be beneficial for well-being either. Dollahite (1998) has convincingly argued that while religious beliefs and practices generally encourage and
promote responsible fathering, some "inner-oriented" forms of spirituality may actually be inimical to fathers' involvement in their children's

lives. Similarly, individualistic, self-oriented spiritual strivings outside of faith-based communities may not be associated with adaptive psychological physical and interpersonal outcomes.

IMPLICATIONS FOR ASSESSING RELIGIOUSNESS

The bulk of psychological research on religion has focused on dispositional traits, measuring individual differences in constructs such as the intrinsic–extrinsic dimension. The limitations of focusing solely at the trait level while relying exclusively on the questionnaire measurement paradigm have been noted (Batson et al., 1992; Gorsuch, 1984). Recall from Chapter 2 that McAdams (1995) distinguishes three levels of personality: dispositional traits (Level I), personal concerns (Level II), and identity or the life narrative (Level III). The bulk of psychological research on religion has focused on Level I, dispositional traits. From this vantage point, religiousness is expressed in broad, decontextualized trans-situational tendencies, such as the intrinsic–extrinsic orientation (Paloutzian, 1996). Researchers examining individual differences in religiousness have emphasized that people are not religious in the same ways. Allport was the first to systematically distinguish between religion as a means to an end (extrinsic) and religion as a way of life (intrinsic). Measures of the former generally show a very different pattern of correlations with criterion variables such as church attendance, prejudice, and mental health than do measures of the latter (Ventis, 1995). As I mentioned earlier in this chapter, even a distinction between intrinsic and extrinsic religiousness, as critical as that is, fails to begin to capture the complexity personal religiosity and spirituality.

Units at Levels II and III, contextualized concerns and identity issues, remain largely unexplored and have much to offer the psychologist interested in religious issues within personality. As Pargament (1992) and others (e.g. Richards & Bergin, 1997) have argued, psychologists need to treat the topic of personal spirituality seriously, since people who report themselves to be motivated spiritually behave and feel differently from those who report other motivations. As the data presented earlier in this chapter testifies, measures of spiritual motivation do contribute significant and unique variance to outcomes that are of central interest to personality and social psychologists.

Moreover, these outcomes are not limited to emotional well-being. Spiritual and religious belief systems usually promise their adherents considerably more than a life of happiness; frequently, in fact, guarantees of emotional bliss or even psychological comfort in the present life are not presented as part of God's ultimate plan. An underlying theme of the following two chapters is that spirituality is associated with much more than emotional well-being. In the next chapter, the role of spirituality in personality integration will be considered. Chapter 7 will consider research examining the ability of spiritual and religious worldviews to provide a sense of meaning and purpose in the face of extreme adversity, and the role of ultimate concerns in the meaning-making process.

CONCLUSIONS

The measurement of spirituality through personal strivings highlights the potential opportunities and challenges for personality researchers interested in how people live lives that are meaningful, valuable, and purpose driven. As we saw in Chapter 3, a number of highly fruitful research programs have provided an empirical foundation for a motivational theory of well-being. Given the research summarized in this chapter the applicability of the goal framework for understanding religion's role in mental and physical health appears equally promising. The inclusion of middle-level units of personality such as strivings into spiritual assessments can complement existing variables and may provide valuable insights into this significant realm of human experience. Moreover, the personal strivings framework offers a conceptual and methodological approach that enables one to examine, using an acceptable scientific framework, spirituality and religiousness within personality.

CHAPTER SIX

From Goal to Whole: Spiritual Strivings and Personality Integration

Difficult however, though it is to save life from fragmentariness,
the penalty for failure is terrific—a harassed, distracted life,
drawn and quartered, that knows no serenity.
—FOSDICK (1943, p. 34)

We have seen in prior chapters how subjective well-being is a function of the possession of and progression toward personally defined, valuable, and meaningful life goals. Yet something more than the singular pursuit of these goals, no matter how "ultimate" they may be, is required for a person to experience a deep and lasting sense of fulfillment and completeness. Life is more than a goal. Our lives are not the sum total of our goals. Without an overall organizational framework that unites separate goal strivings into a coherent structure, a person would have a very difficult time living a life that is meaningful. Baumeister (1991) defines meaning as "a shared mental representation of possible relationships among things, events, and relationships. Thus, meaning *connects* things" (p. 15). As I have contended elsewhere (Emmons, 1996), a goal account of subjective well-being will be painfully incomplete if it fails to deal with the issue of unity, coherence, and integration (or lack thereof) between goals and other aspects of personality. This is not to assume that integration or harmony among the elements of personality is the natural state of affairs nor is necessarily easy to accomplish. Nor does it mean that all patterns that connect are equally

113

healthy. Meaning can be derived from destructive belief systems as well as constructive systems.

As we saw in Chapter 4, conflict and fragmentation are the inevitable by-products of a motivational system. Conflict is a prepotent predictor of distress precisely because it reflects incoherence and disharmony in the personality system. This chapter is devoted to a further explication of the notion of conflict, but now the focus shifts from an emphasis on fragmentation to a focus on integration or unification. The thesis that will be developed here is that personal spirituality is an effective mechanism by which goal integration may be achieved. More generally, the present chapter is concerned with the place of religion within the overall personality. In Chapter 5, the concern was primarily with the effect of religion on personal well-being. What can the personal striving framework contribute to an understanding of the potential role of spirituality in integrated functioning? Is it possible to move from "goal to whole"— from a state of fragmentation to one of relative wholeness? Does spirituality facilitate this movement? Before our discussion is complete, I shall consider the possibility that spiritual striving might also increase fragmentation.

Let us begin by considering what a spiritually oriented lifestyle offers people. Research on the benefits of religion, as discussed in the previous chapter, has focused on the provision of meaning, social and spiritual support, an eternal perspective, hope and happiness, and ultimate acceptance. These may be by-products of a spiritually oriented lifestyle, but at its core, religion offers nothing less than transformation of the person. The objective of religion, of all religions, is that of transformation of the person from fragmentation to integration, from separation to reconciliation. Bringing about unity in the person, rescuing the psyche from inner turmoil and conflict, is the purpose of both theologically and psychologically based interventions. Religion invests human existence with meaning by establishing goals and value systems that pertain to all aspects of a person's life with the potential to confer unity upon disparate experiences (Schimmel, 1997). Faith has been described as "the ongoing weaving of the fabric of life—giving form, order, pattern, cohesion, and holding power to the disparate elements of experience" (Parks, 1993, p. 388). This integration or coherence hypothesis is empirically testable, and a later section of the chapter considers some empirical attempts to examine the association between spiritual strivings and personality integration. An emphasis on integration and wholeness expands the current focus on narrower conceptions of well-being that primarily emphasize personal happiness. At least one study has found that when individuals were asked to explicitly choose between values, desires for meaning, purpose, and freedom from internal conflict were rated as high if not higher than a desire for personal happiness (King & Napa, 1998). Although happiness is generally considered the highest human goal, I will argue in this chapter that personal integrity, as expressed through personality integration, is the sine qua non of effective functioning in life.

GOAL DIFFERENTIATION AND THE SELF

I reviewed the literature on goal characteristics that are predictive of well-being in Chapter 3. A goal parameter with ramifications for well-being that was described in that chapter was the *differentiation* or distinctiveness within one's goal system. Goal differentiation refers to the degree of interrelation that exists between individual goals in the system. A high degree of differentiation exists in systems in which goals are not highly related to each other, and are thus relatively independent. Differentiation as a person characteristic refers to possessing a variety of strivings in a variety of domains. A low degree of differentiation, on the other hand, is characteristic of systems in which the goals are highly related to each other, or are tightly focused upon a singular pursuit. People with relatively undifferentiated goal systems may be either characterized by unity of purpose or fragmentation depending on the degree of coherence among their goals. Differentiation is one component of structural complexity, along with integration (Werner & Kaplan, 1956).

Differentiated striving systems that are poorly integrated are predictive of psychological distress and reactivity. Whether conceptualized in terms of goal conflicts or discrepancies in trait attributes (Donahue et al., 1993), fragmentation is associated with internal as well as external costs. If the self represents a hierarchy of goals that has been "built up, bit by bit, over the years" (Csikszentmihalyi, 1990, p. 34), then goal conflict is indicative of self-fragmentation in the broader sense. Psychic disorder in the form of internal conflict jeopardizes well-being, as the literature reviewed in Chapter 4 unequivocally demonstrated.

Interestingly, a number of different investigators have suggested that linking differentiated, conflicting goals with future positive selves or similar future-oriented mental representations of the self appears to circumvent the deleterious effects of disconnected goals on well-being. Sheldon and Emmons (1995) found that individuals with more links between their goals and future selves, that is, the ability to see one's current intentional action as relating to images of who one wishes to become, may reclaim a sense of successful goal striving. B. R. Little (1993) has linked personal projects with the self by identifying four self-related functions that projects serve: self-expressive (self-defining), self-enhancement (related to self-worth), self-exploration (personal growth), and self-extension (self-transformation). When personal projects are linked to future self-representations, rated progress toward them is higher (Yetim, 1993). King, Richard, and Stemmerich (1998) have documented the importance of people viewing their goals in the context of their larger life story. They found that the strivings that were most predictive of well-being were those that were linked with ultimate life goals and worst fears regarding future life outcomes. Their study signifies the importance of linking proximal goals with future orientations. These research efforts are prime examples of the recent attempt to locate personal goals within a broader framework of personality and identity (Singer & Salovey, 1993) that might facilitate an examination of the mechanisms involved in integration.

From Differentiation to Integration

It is clear from goal research that in order to optimize long-term well-being, people should strive for outcomes which are consistent with the type of person they envision becoming. As we saw in Chapter 4, intrapsychic conflict consistently predicts poor physical and psychological health. Psychological conflicts resulting in the fragmentation of personality are associated with a host of pathological conditions, including poor mental and physical health, disrupted relationships, and decline in cognitive performance (Emmons et al., 1993). Not surprisingly, the writer and practical theologian Harry Emerson Fosdick (1943) said that "occasions when life ceases to be a fraction and becomes an integer are profoundly satisfying" (p. 33). Optimal health and well-being occur when different elements of personality are integrated into a more-or-less coherent whole. Personality integration, defined as "the forging of approximate mental unity out of discordant impulses and aspirations" (Allport, 1950, p. 92), has long been viewed as an important precondition for optimal psychological health. What can the personal strivings framework contribute to an understanding of the processes of personality integration?

The work of Sheldon and Kasser (1995) offers some clues. These researchers attempted to operationalize personality integration and relate it to psychological adjustment. According to Sheldon & Kasser, integration consists of two components: coherence and congruence. Coherence represents the degree to which proximal goals contribute to or are instrumental for longer-term, more distal goals and the degree to which lower-level, subordinate goals are instrumental for higher-level, superordinate strivings; the authors referred to this as "vertical coherence."

Horizontal coherence, on the other hand, occurs when success at particular goals contributes to success at other goals at the same level in the system (goal instrumentality). Congruence involves pursuing goals for self-determined reasons and being oriented toward goals that entail inherently satisfying activity. Congruence in the system occurs when goals are genuinely chosen by the person and fulfill basic needs of autonomy and relatedness. Coherence and congruence were measured through personal strivings. Sheldon and Kasser found that congruence and coherence were related to more favorable levels of subjective health and well-being, to daily measures of mood, vitality, and engagement in meaningful as opposed to distracting activities. A person with a congruent goal system experiences vitality and satisfaction with life; thus, he or she is better able to deal with stress effectively and to perceive daily life events as challenges and opportunities rather than as threats. Self-perceived freedom in striving—or "striving autonomy"—was associated with greater coherence among the different self-attributes. A distinction was made between intrinsic and extrinsic vertical coherence. Intrinsic coherence was based on the degree to which strivings helped bring about the intrinsic values of personal growth, intimacy, and a sense of community; extrinsic coherence was the degree to which strivings helped to bring about financial success, fame, and social recognition. Only intrinsic coherence was related to better psychological functioning.

Given the ubiquity of motivational conflict in everyday life, it becomes imperative to identify conditions that might ameliorate conflict-induced stress and lead to greater harmony, coherence, and integration of personality. Goal-conflict resolution, described in Chapter 4, occurs "when two or more apparently contradictory elements have been transformed into one element that exists without opposition" (Heitler, 1990, p. 5). Although conflicts can be handled as they arise through various attentional mechanisms, long-term resolution requires the establishment of an overarching framework for diverse activities, interests, and goals of the person. One such framework is that which is provided by religion. Personal religious motivation, defined in terms of spiritual, goals, beliefs, and values, is hypothesized by psychologists (e.g., Allport, 1950; Ellison & Smith, 1991) and theologians (e.g., Tillich, 1957) to serve as a central integrating and organizing force in people's lives. Religion is all-encompassing and embraces all of life (Schimmel, 1997); it thus has the potential to forge unity and coherence out of chaos and fragmentation. Batson et al. (1992) wrote that religion "has a coherence that goes beyond a collection of beliefs, attitudes, emotions, and behaviors. It seems to combine and transcend these . . . providing a sense of integrity" (p. 7). Before we examine the empirical literature, however, let us consider psychological and theological perspectives on personal integration.

RELIGION AND PERSONALITY
INTEGRATION: THEORY

Both theological and psychological perspectives on personality integration have been in existence for some time. As Jeeves (1997) and Myers (1978) have argued, theological and psychological explanations of behavioral phenomena should not be seen as competing or conflicting, but rather as providing complementary accounts at differing levels of analysis. Personality integration offers one of the best illustrations of how theological perspectives might augment psychological levels of analysis.

Contributions from Personality Theory

According to several personality theorists, the hallmark of the psychologically healthy person is integration. Lester (1995) provides an overview of the concept of integration within theories of personality. One of the best-known formulations is that of Angyal (1941), who considered life to be a constant process of balancing the need for self-expansion, which he called the striving for autonomy, with the need for connectedness, which he called the striving for homonomy. Healthy personality development involves the constant synthesis of these opposing tendencies without allowing one set of strivings to achieve prepotence over the other. Neurotic symptoms are the result of magnification of one tendency and minimization of the other. Angyal did not explicitly address the role of religion in the integration of these motivational forces, but his contemporary, Klein (1944), emphasized "the integrative striving that underlies all religious life. Striving is the basic human trait; religious striving is the ultimate expression of this trait" (cited in Vande Kemp, 1995, p. 205).

The ability of religion to confer upon personality a unifying philosophy of life was perhaps the central theme of Allport's (1950) book titled *The Individual and His Religion*, which has been dubbed a "masterpiece" in the psychology of religion (Kelly, 1995). In keeping with his general emphasis on healthy psychological functioning in personality, Allport was primarily interested in mature expressions of personal religiousness. In his view, mature religion is not a compartmentalized sphere of life but rather is comprehensive and integrally related to the rest of life. Allport (1950) was impressed by the coherence and integration in personality that personal religion can foster: "The religious sentiment . . . is the portion of personality that arises at the core of the life and is directed toward the infinite. It has the longest range intentions, and for this reason is capable of conferring marked integration upon personality. . . . It is man's ultimate attempt to enlarge and to complete his own personality" (p. 142). It is the comprehensiveness of religion, in contrast with other belief systems, that is believed to account for the ability of the religious sentiment to forge a harmonious pattern out of a patchwork of discordant impulses and strivings.

Conflict and Integration: Theological Contributions

The prevalence of conflicting forces in people's lives has long been recognized in theological writings. The New Testament writer Paul knew well in his own life the nature of such inner turmoil. In his letter to the Romans, Paul spoke of finding himself unable to do what he wants to do, yet finding himself doing that which he does not want to do. Similarly, Martin Luther (1525/1957), the father of the Protestant Reformation, spoke of the "bondage of the will," and St. Augustine's (397/1960) depictions of his internal fragmentation as "a house divided" in his autobiographical *Confessions* are legendary. To be divided is to lack integrity. Indeed, the word "integrity" comes from the same root as "integrate," which means to achieve wholeness. Internal division or fragmentation is the opposite of integrity. To be a person of integrity is to be a person who is whole, who is steadfast in conviction in deed and in word. In his New Testament epistle, James encourages believers to be people of integrity: "When will you ever learn that 'believing' is useless without doing what God wants you to? Faith that does not result in good deeds is not real faith" (James 2:20, *The Living Bible*, 1988). In the Chinese Taoist tradition, health and longevity depend upon balance and harmony among The Three Treasures: essence, energy, and spirit (Reid, 1994). Buddhism teaches that ideal development involves a blending of integrated individuality with the harmony underlying the cosmos.

It is also highly instructive to consider the meaning of the term "religion," which comes from the Latin *religio*, meaning to bind or connect. In our bodies, ligaments connect tissues that hold our bones and internal organs in place. Religion is similarly a binding force, with the potential to unite and bind internal fragmentation. Religion can produce connections at three levels: (1) internally—providing an integrated set of beliefs, intentions and actions, (2) horizontally—between people through a shared identity within a faith community, and (3) vertically—to creation and the Creator. The root meaning of the Hebrew word *shalom*, which appears over 250 times in the Scriptures, includes the concepts of wholeness, completeness, and harmony. *Shalom* is the integrated state of a person who is in a right relationship with God, with others, and within him- or herself (Ellison & Smith, 1991). It is the inner serenity of being harmoniously at peace within and without. Ellison and Smith (1991) provide a excellent overview of the meaning of the term "integration" within a psychotheological framework. A psychotheological portrait views the person as an integrated system "functioning as God intended" (p. 36).

In previous chapters I have drawn heavily upon Paul Tillich's concept of faith as ultimate concern. The relation of ultimate concern to the rest of personality concerned Tillich greatly, and was a major part of his 1957 book. For Tillich, faith is an "act of centering." It is the centered movement of the whole personality toward something of ultimate meaning and significance. I repeat the quotation from Tillich: "The ultimate concern gives depth, direction, and unity to all other concerns, and with them, to the whole personality" (p. 105). His position cannot be stated strongly enough, or reiterated frequently enough. He described ultimate concern as a "passionate concern," as the "ground of everything that is," as "related to all sides of reality," as that which "unites all elements of man's personal life, the bodily, the unconscious, the conscious, the spiritual ones" (p. 106). The capacity to go beyond immediate and preliminary concerns is what gives life meaning, according to Tillich. Without ultimate concern, Tillich goes on to say, both the external world and internal workings of the mind conspire to produce a state of "complete disintegration" (p. 107). It has been suggested that the term "ultimate concern" is Tillich's abstract translation of Jesus' great commandment: "Love the Lord your God with all your heart and with all your soul and with all your mind" (Matthew 22:37, NIV).

Contemporary theologian J. I. Packer (1993) states that the ultimate purpose in life is to know God: "What makes life worthwhile is having a big enough objective, something which catches the imagination and lays hold of our allegiance . . . what higher, more exalted, and more compelling goal can there be than to know God?" (p. 34). In the Geneva Catechism John Calvin (1559/1984) declared that the "ultimate goal of life, the chief end of man, is to glorify God and to enjoy him forever" (p. 108). In his classic The Christian Life, Calvin (1559/1984) stated his belief that as God's own people, every part of our existence should be directed to him as the only legitimate goal. If knowing God is the ultimate goal in life, and one lives life with that unifying philosophy, all of the other preliminary desires, goals, concerns, wishes, and strivings will fall into place. To paraphrase Oxford University professor and theologian C. S. Lewis (1960), if God is at the hub of people's lives, the spokes of the wheel cannot other than be at perfect alignment with each other. These are powerful statements, which from a scientific vantage point lack truth value in the absence of empirical corroboration. In principle such claims are testable by examining the presence of the divine in people's self-reported goal strivings. What little relevant research there is suggests that people often report that inner harmony and wholeness replace inner turmoil and fragmentation following spiritual conversion, the topic to which we now turn.

RELIGION AND PERSONALITY
INTEGRATION: RESEARCH

Before describing some recent attempts by my colleagues and myself to assess personality integration through personal strivings, other efforts to study this association should be acknowledged. In their review of over 100 articles on religion and mental health, Batson et al. (1992) identified seven components of mental health, one of which was "personality unification and organization." Only 1 of the 115 studies was relevant to this conception of mental health, and its results were inconclusive. The authors concluded that there was no clear relationship between personality unification and religious involvement "because virtually no relevant data exist" (p. 255).

In a study that has not received much attention in the psychology of religion literature, Sacks (1979) examined the effect of spiritual exercises of Saint Ignatius of Loyola on integration of the self-concept. In a sample of 50 Jesuit novices, he found that a 4-week period of secluded meditation resulted in a significant increase in self-integration, as measured by Loevinger's (1976) concept of ego development. Little detail is provided about the nature of the spiritual exercises, making it difficult to isolate the specific cause of the increase in cognitive integration. Evidently, though, the 30-day exercise sufficiently increased these men's ability to assimilate conflicting self-representations into a unified self-system. Unfortunately, there is no information on how long the effect lasted beyond the period of observation. The uniqueness of the sample also makes generalizability problematic.

Using a very different definition of integration, a more recent study by Blaine and Trivedi (1997) found that one's definition of religiousness matters in the link between integration and religiousness. These researchers found that evaluative complexity of the self-concept, or the extent to which positive and negative self-descriptions are connected in memory, is related to the religious quest dimension of religious orientation, but not to a global measure of religious belief strength. Moreover, they present data showing that evaluative complexity helps buffer individuals from depression. In another study, Blaine, Trivedi, and Eshleman (1998) examined the link between strength of religious beliefs and self-concept certainty and positivity. Self-concept certainty is an indicator of integrated functioning and was found to mediate the relationship between religiousness and well-being. Furthermore, religion appeared to integrate self-aspects even in nonreligious knowledge domains—for example, in interpersonal and work domains. Religious belief systems, according to Blaine et al. operate as integrative frameworks.

Conflict and Religious Conversion

Internal conflict as an impetus for religious conversion is a hypothesis that has achieved nearly the status of dogma in the psychology of religion. Stratton (1911) first put forth the thesis that personal religiousness is rooted in internal conflict. Emotional distress in the form of intense personal conflict is frequently cited as a precursor that precedes and paves the way for conversion. In reviewing the factors operating in conversion, Clark (1958) concluded that "the most basic psychological element in conversion would appear to be conflict . . . the attraction of two incompatible ways of life" (p. 202). Arguably the most famous case of religious conversion in history was that of St. Augustine (397/1960), the bishop of Hippo, in North Africa. His internal battles between the forces of light and darkness and their ultimate resolution through identification with Christ are graphically documented in his autobiography, required reading for students of spiritual formation. Clark's (1958) classic psychology of religion text devotes an entire chapter to religious conflict. He argues that while conflict plays a part in all personal growth, it does so especially in religious growth. By forcing a choice between values, religious frameworks and worldviews may succeed in reducing day-to-day conflict between competing choices. After all, if one sees parenting as a divinely sanctioned activity, as described in Chapter 5, the tendency to experience conflict between work and family activities is likely to be significantly reduced. In what is regarded by many as the landmark work on psychology and religion, William James (1902) stated, "To experience religion . . . is the process by which a self hitherto divided and consciously wrong inferior and unhappy, becomes unified and consciously right superior and happy, in consequence of its firmer hold upon religious realities" (p. 157). James also devoted an entire chapter of *The Varieties of Religious Experience* to the nature of the divided self and the process of unification. Both James and Clark suggest that psychology has replaced theological notions of redemption and salvation with the psychological concerns of integration and unification, echoing the parallels I drew earlier between theologically and psychologically based modes of healing. In the biblical perspective, people as sinners are struggling for redemption; in psychological perspectives, fragmented persons are seeking integration and self-consistency. This parallel is expressed eloquently by Allport (1950): "Religion and therapy are alike in their insistence upon the need for greater unification and order in personality.

Both recognize that the healthy mind requires a hierarchical organization of sentiments, ordinarily with one master sentiment holding the dominant position. In principle, the religious interest, being the most comprehensive, is best able to serve as an integrative agent" (p. 79).

Although not involving religious conversion per se, the fascinating study of quantum life changes reported by Miller and C'deBaca (1994) should be mentioned here. Their study was an intensive examination of 55 people reporting major transformations in personality (primarily in value hierarchies). Transformations were defined in terms of value shifts, with the majority of participants reporting an increase in intrinsically spiritual values, such as forgiveness, humility, and God's will, and a decline in the importance of extrinsic values such as attractiveness, popularity, and wealth. A number of experiences gave rise to these "quantum changes," only a small percentage of which might be considered religious or spiritual in origin. The authors offer "value conflict" as a possible mechanism for change, suggesting that perceived discrepancies between sincerely held values or between values and actual behaviors might serve as a catalyst for personality change.

Trauma and Spiritual Conversion

Research on coping with trauma has shown that religion can enable people to put their lives back together following catastrophes. Trauma is a personality disintegrator (Epstein, 1991), it shatters belief systems, results in loss of meaning, and destroys relationships. Religion ideally reconnects the person to others through a socially supportive faith community and aids in the restoration of meaning. It has been said that trauma produces either religious conversion or mental illness (although some would argue that those are one and the same). Boisen (1936), in his *Explorations of the Inner World*, drew a parallel between psychopathology and religious experience. As existential conditions, both religious conversion and mental illness are seen as processes of disorganization and reorganization and transformation of personality. In his description of the implications of Boisen's perspective, Pruyser (1960) proposes that another common link between psychopathology and conversion is that each deal with "human potentiality and ultimate loyalties" (p. 119). Trauma was one of the most common potentiating events for quantum change in Miller and C'deBaca's (1994) sample.

Despite the spiritual literature being replete with anecdotal reports and persuasive individual cases of wholeness brought about by conversion, there exists no systematic, rigorous research on whether religious conversion can truly bring about integration or wholeness of personality. A priority for future research should be longitudinal studies, employing pre- and post-conversion measures of personality integration. Only then will researchers be able to draw solid conclusions from what remains a fascinating yet systematically unexplored thesis. Also, various meanings of conversion need to be delineated. For example, the deepening or intensification of faith might not be considered conversion in the usual sense of the term, but such changes can lead to increasing self-integration. Religious change in Eastern traditions might be better captured by the term "enlightenment" rather than conversion, and the attainment of enlightenment through meditative techniques is geared toward increasing self-integration through the loss of the self (Brown, 1993).

Before leaving this section on conversion, one recent exemplary study on conversion needs to be described. Zinnbauer and Pargament (1998) compared inner changes in identity in spiritual converts with nonconverts who increased in their religious faith gradually, and with religious individuals who had not experienced a recent change in their faith. Participants were also asked to what degree they felt that their religious or spiritual change had redirected their goals. Compared to the other two groups, the converts were more likely to report a positive life transformation, as reflected in a more unified sense of self and a belief that their goals had become more significant and meaningful. To my knowledge, this was the first empirical study that attempted to examine transformational changes in goals as a function of religious life change.

Spiritual Strivings and Personality Integration

The literature review suggests that there is reason to believe that personal religious motivation will facilitate personality integration, thus reducing the pernicious effect of conflict on mental and physical health. In a recent study, Chi Cheung, Keivan Tehrani, and I (Emmons, Cheung, & Tehrani, 1998) tested the hypothesis that religiousness or spirituality can serve as an integrating framework which reduces the overall amount of conflict within a person's goal system and fosters coherence in personality. The relationship between spiritual strivings and personality integration was assessed through measures of goal coherence (Sheldon & Kasser, 1995). A goal-based approach to integration offers several advantages. The terms "wholeness," "integration," "congruence," and "coherence" and related concepts are used quite frequently in the health psychology popular literature, and thus there is a strong need for clear conceptual and methodological clarity. In order to advance both research and interventions on spiritual factors in wholeness and healing, there is a strong need for methodological rigor. Applying established technologies for assessing personal goal concerns could lead to some progress in the study of spirituality and personal integration.

Seventy-eight adults were administered the Personal Striving Assessment Packet in which at least 10 personal goals were generated and appraised on a series of rating scales. Spirituality in striving content was coded using three of the criteria from the Emmons, Cheung, and Tehrani (1998) study, described in the last chapter: relational/affective (e.g., "Get closer to God"), cognitive or belief-based (e.g., "Increase my understanding of God"), and behavioral-ritual (e.g., "Pray daily"). Overall integration was assessed via the Striving Instrumentality Matrix, in which participants made pairwise comparisons between each pair of strivings for the degree to which each striving facilitates or impedes progress toward the other striving. A global striving conflict index was created by summing the individual ratings for each goal. Two other integration measures were derived from the appraisal dimensions. Ambivalence was assessed by asking how much unhappiness would be felt upon successful consummation of the goal (Emmons & King, 1988), and interpersonal conflict was assessed by asking participants to rate the degree of interpersonal strain the striving produces in their everyday interactions. All striving integration measures possess adequate reliability and validity (Emmons & King, 1988; Sheldon & Kasser, 1995). Each of these measures should be considered proxys for integration. Obviously, it is not possible to do justice to the profound concept of "personal integration" in any one empirical study, or even a program of studies. It is also possible to be a highly integrated person and still experience conflict in daily goal pursuits.

Following the striving assessment, a number of questionnaire measures of conflict were administered. These included the Ambivalence Over Expressing Religiousness Questionnaire (ARQ), a 25 item-scale that measures conflicts relating to the communication of religious beliefs, the Beliefs About Conflict Scale (BACS), which assesses subjective beliefs about the (in)compatibility of various life domains (e.g., family and work) and the conflict items from the Religious Quest Scale (Kojetin, McIntosh, Bridges, & Spilka, 1987). The ARQ was patterned after the Ambivalence Over Expressing Emotion Questionnaire described in Chapter 4, and sample items include "I want to openly express my religious beliefs, but I am afraid that others will get the wrong impression of me," and "Often I'd like to share with others what God has done in my life, but something seems to be holding me back." All of these measures can be considered indicators of "horizontal coherence," to use Sheldon and Kasser's (1995) terminology, in that they reflect instrumental or conflictual relations between personality elements at a similar level of abstraction.

Pearson correlations were computed between the proportion of spiritual strivings from each person's total number of strivings and each measure of integration. Nineteen percent of all strivings were coded as spiritual, and 6% of all strivings mentioned God or Jesus Christ. A composite measure of integration was created by first standardizing, and then summing the six integration measures. These correlations are shown in Table 6.1. Overall goal conflict was significantly negatively associated with both spiritual strivings ($p < .01$) and theistic (those in which explicit reference to God is made, see Table 6.2) strivings ($p < .01$).

Both measures of spiritual striving were negatively related to scores on the Quest conflict scale ($p < .01$). The overall composite integration measure correlated positively and significantly with spiritual and theistic strivings ($p < .05$). None of the other four measures of conflict were related to the two striving indices. In all, 4 out of 12 correlations were statistically significant, including a standardized composite measure of integration. In addition, t-tests revealed that spiritual and theistic strivings produced overall less conflict (hence greater integration) compared with nonspiritual and nontheistic strivings ($p < .01$).

It might be argued here that there is nothing unique about spiritual strivings in bringing about a reduction of overall goal conflict. Perhaps a concentration of goals in any domain would be sufficient to produce less overall systemic conflict. To examine this possibility, we examined each of 10 other striving categories, including achievement, intimacy, affiliation, and power. The percentage of strivings in each of these domains

TABLE 6.1. Correlations between Integration Measures and Spiritual and Theistic Strivings

Integration measure	Spiritual strivings	Theistic strivings
Striving Conflict	−.52**	−.39**
Striving Ambivalence	.00	.12
Interpersonal Strain	−.01	.00
ARQ	.13	.02
BACS	.19	.20
Quest–conflict	−.33**	−.35**
Composite Integration	.25*	.20*

Note. ARQ, Ambivalence Over Expressing Religiousness Questionnaire; BACS, Beliefs About Conflict Scale: Quest–conflict, Religious Quest Scale, conflict subscale. $N = 78$.
*$p < .05$; **$p < .01$.

TABLE 6.2. Examples of Theistic Strivings

"Be pleasing to God in all that I do each day."

"Glorify God."

"Love God with my whole heart."

"Understand God's will."

"Understand and perceive God in the world."

"Live my religion and grow closer to God."

"Glorify God with my life."

"Know that God loves me for who I am and try to love others the same way."

"Be faithful in stewardship of what God has provided."

"Seek the Lord's guidance for the day."

"Look for the Lord's blessings in life."

"Believe the Lord has a plan for my life."

"Live a godly life."

"Take time for God."

failed to correlate with our measures of integration. Thus, spiritual strivings are uniquely associated with overall goal integration.

The Striving Instrumentality matrices of two of the participants in the Emmons and Cheung study are shown in Figure 6.1. It can be seen that the top participant had absolutely no conflict between his strivings and perfect positive instrumentality, a highly unusual profile. Seventy percent of his strivings were theistic, compared to an average of 6% for the sample. The profile of the second participant reveals that the striving to "Share my faith with others" produced strain with three of her other goals, including "Keep contact with family" and "Treat others with love."

The results of the Emmons, Cheung, and Tehrani (1998) study provide preliminary support for the thesis expressed earlier by Tillich, Allport, and James, among others. Greater levels of spiritual strivings, whether measured at relatively broad or narrow levels, tend to be associated with less overall conflict within a person's goal system, and thus a greater degree of integration. A goal-theoretical perspective is a means of examining integrative personality processes. It should also be stressed here that the concept of personality integration, much like the concept of spirituality itself, is a broad, diffuse concept that cannot be easily reduced to a pat definition and certainly not operationalized in any kind of comprehensive way through a few self-report measures. Although we cannot do the concept of integration justice here, there does appear to be sufficient evidence to warrant continued examination of the thesis that religion can serve as a unifier and integrator of personality.

ID _____

Striving Instrumentality Matrix

STRIVINGS		merge my will in...	love God	praise God...	enjoy God's...	love all of...	bring God's creatures...	fulfill relig...	commune w/ God	seek the good...	serve humanity	
		1	2	3	4	5	6	7	8	9	10	
merge my will in God's pleasure	1		+2	+2	+2	+2	+2	+2	+2	+2	+2	45
love God	2	+2		+2	+2	+2	+2	+2	+2	+2	+2	45
praise God in action & thought	3	+2	+2		+2	+2	+2	+2	+2	+2	+2	45
enjoy God's world	4	+2	+2	+2		+2	+2	+2	+2	+2	+2	45
love all of God's creatures	5	+2	+2	+2	+2		+2	+2	+2	+2	+2	45
bring God's creatures closer to God	6	+2	+2	+2	+2	+2		+2	+2	+2	+2	45
fulfill religious obligations	7	+2	+2	+2	+2	+2	+2		+2	+2	+2	45
commune with God	8	+2	+2	+2	+2	+2	+2	+2		+2	+2	45
seek the good in all things	9	+2	+2	+2	+2	+2	+2	+2	+2		+2	45
serve humanity	10	+2	+2	+2	+2	+2	+2	+2	+2	+2		45

ID _____

Striving Instrumentality Matrix

ID	STRIVINGS		Treat others w/ love	Share my faith	Spend time w/ God	Please my boyfriend	Do my best in school	Spend time w/ friends	Exercise Regularly	Keep contact w/ family	Eat healthy	Take a sabbath	
			1	2	3	4	5	6	7	8	9	10	
12	Treat others with love	1		+2	0	+2	0	+2	0	+2	0	0	35
13	Share my faith with others	2	-1		0	0	0	-1	0	-2	0	0	23
03	Spend time with God	3	+2	+2		+2	+2	+2	+2	+2	+2	+2	45
02	Please my boyfriend	4	+1	0	0		0	-1	0	0	0	1	26
01	Do my best in school	5	0	0	0	0		-2	7	0	0	0	23
04	Spend time with friends	6	+2	+1	0	0	0		-1	0	-2	-1	26
05	Exercise Regularly	7	0	0	0	0	+0	0		0	+1	0	29
11	Keep contact w/ family	8	+1	0	0	-1	0	0	0		0	0	27
14	Eat healthy	9	0	0	0	0	0	0	+1	0		0	28
15	Take a sabbath	10	+2	+1	+2	0	0	0	0	0	0		32

FIGURE 6.1. Striving instrumentality matrices of participants high in integration and in spiritual strivings.

Spiritual Interventions and Integration

While these initial results are encouraging, the relations between spirituality and integration need to be explored more systematically, in a diverse range of populations and using a variety of rigorously developed measures of integration. Furthermore, goal-based units have been shown to be effective in therapeutic interventions. Therapeutic techniques through which people gain control over consciousness and thus reduce internal conflicts constitute an agenda for future research. What are the mechanisms by which order and harmony in consciousness can be achieved? Successful resolution requires three sequential processes (Greenberg & Safran, 1987): (1) an initial expression of the incompatibilities between the different components (opposition phase); (2) awareness and experiencing of feelings associated with both sides, including taking full responsibility for these feelings (merging phase); and (3) integration of the conflicting sides (integration phase). It might be profitable to assess changes in internal goal conflicts as a function of spiritually based intervention techniques such as prayer, meditation, or other spiritual practices such as those in the Sacks (1979) study. Studying persons who are especially disciplined in awareness training that transforms consciousness ought to facilitate understanding the perceptual reorganization that conflict resolution requires.

In Chapter 3, I introduced "Sissy," a 23-year-old female whose strivings were dominated by unrealistic strivings for perfection and total approval and acceptance. How might an infusion of spiritual concern transform her concerns into goals that allow for greater purpose, meaning, and satisfaction? The target for intervention would be her unrealistic goals involving unattainable states in relationships with fallible human beings. Propst (1988) describes several techniques for transforming consciousness that are particularly effective in dealing with perfectionistic strivers such as Sissy. Two essential ingredients of this spiritual framework for counseling are self-dialogue and the gaining of a transcendent, divine perspective in viewing the self. Self-dialogue, according to Propst, begins with self-examination, whereby we learn to view ourselves outside of our relationships to each other and see ourselves more as God sees us. Drawing on the relational theologies of as Reinhold Niebuhr, Karl Barth, and Emil Brunner, Propst stresses that a search for the perfect relationship be replaced with a relationship with the divine, where a person is free to be truly him- or herself and thus enable others to be themselves. Affirmation from God relieves us of the burden of basing our self-definitions on other's reactions to us. The freedom that this new perspective grants is beautifully depicted in the following passage from Tillich (1948): "You are accepted. You are accepted, accepted by that which is greater than you, and the name of which you do not know. Do not ask for the name now; perhaps you will find it later. Do not try to do anything now, perhaps later you will do much. Do not seek for anything, do not perform anything, do not intend anything. Simply accept the fact that you are accepted" (pp. 155–156). Propst (1988) provides concrete illustrations examples of how the transformation of underlying assumptions about the self can result in a new life, replacing a life of fragmentation and despair with one of wholeness and inner security. One can only speculate on how Sissy's strivings to "Be accepted by everyone," "Perform at perfection at my job," "Gain the approval of my father," and "Appear together all the time" might be influenced by the confrontation with some of these cognitive restructuring techniques within a spiritual framework. Obviously, a religiously based framework will not be appropriate for everyone, but, when it is, it can be a powerful adjunct to secular-based therapies.

Mechanisms Linking Spirituality with Personality Integration

How does a commitment to self-transcendent, intrinsically meaningful goals foster personal wholeness? What are some potential explanations for why spirituality may foster coherence and integration of personality? Spiritual strivings tend to be located at a higher level of the self-regulatory system than are other goals, and according to control theory (Carver & Scheier, 1998), regulating one's behavior with regard to higher-order abstract principles leads to greater consistency. Spiritual strivings are also likely to meet basic organismic needs for self-transcendence, and thus are likely to be inherently satisfying and growth-promoting (Sheldon & Kasser, 1995).

The identification of mechanisms by which spirituality promotes health are only beginning to be understood. The Emmons, Cheung, and Tehrani (1998) study suggests that spirituality fosters optimal health through a reduction of overall conflict, in that a commitment to a spiritually oriented lifestyle is one factor that appears to facilitate congruence, integration, and wholeness of the person. Perhaps religious beliefs and experience promote congruence between the analytical/rational and holistic/experiential information-processing systems (Epstein, 1994). Epstein presents compelling evidence for the operation of these two different conceptual systems of the mind, and argues that "religion provides perhaps the most impressive evidence of all that there are two fundamentally different modes of processing information" (p. 712).

Two additional mechanisms by which spirituality might enhance well-being are through the provision of social support (McIntosh, Silver,

& Wortman, 1993) and spiritual support (Maton, 1989). Horizontal and vertical connectedness provide not only valuable coping resources, but also knowledge that, even with all of one's flaws and imperfections, one is unconditionally accepted. This insight can free one from the overreliance on others or material possessions as validators of self-worth. With this knowledge comes the ability to genuinely enter into relationships and to enjoy all of the benefits of social support that come from healthy interpersonal relations. At times spirituality may, however, lead to interpersonal conflict, as in marital religious heteronomy. Negative support is, in fact, a stronger predictor of health outcomes than is positive support (Rook, 1984). Future research should examine negative religious or spiritual support. One way to do this in a goal framework is to examine perceived hindrance of spiritual goal attainment (Brunstein et al., 1996; Ruehlman & Wolchik, 1988).

To function in accordance with our inner nature, our goals and purposes must be in harmony with each other. To return to C. S. Lewis's analogy, even if we successfully accomplish goal after goal, unless we have these goals aligned with each other like spokes on a wheel, our physical, mental, and interpersonal lives will suffer. Through connecting vertically to the divine, it may be possible to connect intrapsychically as well. In an argument rooted in the Zeigarnik effect, Allport (1950) contended that goals which are never quite fulfilled are best able to direct attention, guide current striving, and maintain unity. Religion thus constitutes the most effective form of integration said Allport, because religious strivings, more than any other, are never fully realized, never completely attained: "Because religious accomplishment is always incomplete, its cementing character in the personal life is therefore all the greater" (p. 93).

RELIGION AS INCREASING
PERSONALITY FRAGMENTATION

An explicit assumption of the work described in this chapter is that religion and spirituality generally promote integrated personal functioning. The optimistic tone of the chapter should not be interpreted as suggesting that religion always acts to enhance integrated functioning. Before leaving the topic of religion and personality integration, we should consider the contexts under which spirituality and religious striving might actually increase conflict and fragmentation rather than reduce it. Doubt and conflict are a normal part of spiritual development, as many authors have pointed out. As conflict is a normal part of growth, including religious growth, spiritually oriented lifestyles can be associated with more rather than less conflict. Such conflict need not be detrimental to one's well-being, though in reality it often is. Religious strivings might make people aware of discrepancies between what they believe and what they actually do (the faith versus practice gap). Although ideally such discrepancies can be motivating and lead to enhanced striving and ultimately to deeper faith, discrepancies between belief and action can also engender powerful feelings of inappropriate guilt, depression, and self-recrimination.

Internal religious conflict as well as religious strivings themselves can take their toll in a variety of ways on interpersonal relationships. From the beginning of time, religious differences between people have produced conflicts of varying magnitudes, ranging from physical avoidance to physical confrontation. In daily life, people may be reluctant to express their personal religion for fear of offending others with different beliefs. Research has shown that within marriages, religious homonomy is a predictor of marital adjustment, whereas religious heteronomy predicts marital dissatisfaction (Call & Heaton, 1997). Strongly held convictions coupled with strong taboos against their expression can result in powerful conflicts.

The strivings framework for the study of spirituality might be able to shed some light on how and why religion can cause problems in life functioning. One of the strivings of the participant whose goals are shown in the lower half of Figure 6.1 is "Share my faith with others." It appears to produce considerable conflict for this subject's life, as it is perceived as having a harmful effect on "Treat others with love," "Spend time with friends," and "Keep in contact with family." Conflict is a subjective experience; we do not know why for this individual that a life of faith is unintegrated with other valuable strivings. Perhaps the religious strivings were communicated with a dogmatic arrogance rather than out of loving concern. More effective communication skills, a greater sensitivity to other's beliefs, or a greater humility regarding one's own religious views might each be valuable skills to cultivate, serving to reduce some of the intrapsychic conflict for this person.

GENERATIVITY AS SPIRITUALITY

Spirituality and integration may also be viewed from the lens of generativity theory. Nearly 50 years ago Erikson (1950) introduced the concept of generativity into his lifespan theory of human development. Generativity is a concern for guiding and promoting the next generation through parenting, as well as through teaching, mentoring, and generating products that will survive the self and contribute positively to the next generation (Erikson, 1950; McAdams & de St. Aubin, 1992; Snarey, 1993). Erikson first introduced the concept of generativity as the seventh and longest stage of his eight-stage theory of psychosocial development throughout the life cycle. During the majority of the adult years, "generativity versus stagnation" is thought to assume a central role in the human psyche. According to Erikson, adults in the generative stage are able to expand their focus beyond themselves and intimate partners toward caring for future generations. Generativity is manifested both privately and publicly, as an inner desire whose realization may promote healthy development and psychological and physical well-being. From a societal perspective, generativity is a valuable resource that "may undergird social institutions, encourage citizen's contributions and commitments to the public good, motivate efforts to sustain continuity from one generation to the next, and initiate social change" (McAdams & de St. Aubin, 1998). Although generative concern is often expressed through parenthood, it is not limited to that realm. One may be generative in a variety of contexts, including work and professional activities, volunteerism, neighborhood and community activism, religious and political organizations, and involvement in environmental causes.

Although generativity has recently come to the attention of psychologists, sociologists, and historians, its utility for understanding the spirituality of everyday life, or what Rubinstein (1994) has referred to as "pragmatic spirituality," has yet to be developed. Seldom does the literature on generativity mention that it is a profoundly spiritual construct, particularly likely to be imbued with spiritual significance in persons without a conventional religious ideology or institutional affiliation. There are several reasons for associating generativity with spirituality. Generativity is believed to be rooted in a desire for symbolic immortality (Lifton, 1979), a desire to symbolically defy death by creating a legacy that both extends and outlives the self. Central to both generativity and spirituality is the idea of transcending the self. Self-transcendence draws adults out of their self-preoccupation and connects them to higher powers, other people, institutions, and broader societal and global concerns. As Rubinstein (1994) has persuasively argued, symbolic immortality cannot be achieved in isolation, but instead requires self-transcending structures. Several facets of generativity, including loving and caring for future generations, concerns with the nature of personal finitude, belief in the fundamental goodness and worthwhileness of human life, and concern for the well-being of others suggest the presence of a spiritual component. Dollahite, Slife, and Hawkins (1997) also discuss the spiritual aspects of generativity. They approach generativity from a family perspective, and view generativity as "inherently spiritual, because in our definition it involves transcending selfishness, the demands of the present, and the attractions and distractions of one's own generation" (p. 469). Generative acts are often imbued with a sacred component, continue the authors, using the language of sanctification that was described in Chapter 5.

Generativity and Personality Integration

Generativity may foster personality integration of the type with which this chapter is concerned. Singer and Salovey (1993) conceive of personal strivings as thumbnail sketches of generativity scripts. They comment that "the long-term goals that we acknowledge as playing a role in what we are typically trying to do are really statements to ourselves about how we want the plot of our life stories to turn out" (p. 79). Stories are what provide purpose, unity, and structure to lives, according to McAdams's (1993) life story model of identity. Somewhat paradoxically, generativity requires both self-aggrandizing and self-sacrificing behavior, either of which, in extreme and unmitigated form, can be a risk factor for physical illness. Generative commitments and strivings seemingly offer the person a vehicle for self-transcendence while simultaneously satisfying the need for symbolic immortality. Thus, generativity, or what we are calling pragmatic spirituality, may solve the dilemma between individualistic pursuit and broader and deeper societal concern, reconciling the need for independence with the need for intimacy, or harmonizing the strivings toward autonomy and homonomy, according to Angyal (1941).

The pervasive relationship between conflict and psychological and physical dysfunction may be relevant to the findings that generativity strivings are related to higher levels of well-being. According to McAdams (1993; McAdams & de St. Aubin, 1992), generativity involves the creative blending, or coalescing, of intimacy and power motivation. Generativity involves both creating and giving up a product, and surrendering control. These two processes represent an agentic as well as an intimate act. To quote McAdams (1989): "Generativity challenges us to be both powerful and intimate, expansive and surrendering at the same time. In motivational terms, generativity draws on our desire to be strong and our desire to be close to others, mandating that we integrate and reconcile power and intimacy motivation" (p. 163). Through the creative integration of agentic and communal needs, the generative individual is able to override the potential for conflict between these two motivational themes, thus achieving a reconciliation of the often-competing needs for power and intimacy. As a form of "pragmatic spirituality," generativity may facilitate integration among not only the fundamental needs described by Angyal and McAdams, but also among other elements of the self.

RELIGION AND THE CONSTRUCTION
OF IDENTITY

The answer to the question "Who am I?" takes on a different meaning for a person operating within a religious or spiritual worldview. Recall that in McAdams's (1995) tripartite framework of the person, Level III concerns how persons make sense of who they are in the world, and how they create life stories that provide their lives with overall unity, meaning, and purpose. Religious considerations play a major role in this level of personality, as people construct a life story often rooted in a religious ideology that gives a unique meaning to their life. Along those lines, Beit-Hallahmi (1989) argues that religion is an identity-maintenance system, providing a bridge between individualistic and collectivist identities. In several collections of life stories (Colby & Damon, 1992; Franz & Stewart, 1994; McAdams, 1993) spirituality as a guiding, integrating, and empowering force is a recurring theme. Religious narratives function as potent identity stories in the diverse lives of these men and women. Conversion narratives in the form of the personal testimony are a powerful means of consolidating and strengthening one's new religious identity (Beit-Hallahmi, 1989; Rambo, 1993; Stromberg, 1993). McAdams (1996) notes that the use of metaphor is a defining feature of personal identity. The richness of metaphor that religious systems provide (e.g., viewing major life changes such as divorce and remarriage as involving the death and burial of an old life and a resurrection to a new one) may be a potent means of constructing identity (Atkinson, 1995; Rambo, 1993) and thus are ideally suited to story-based methodologies.

As the problem of identity is the problem of constructing unity, purpose, and coherence in one's life, religion may offer a particularly compelling pathway for many. The general message of this chapter has been that religion or spirituality can provide a unifying philosophy of life and serve as an integrating and stabilizing force in the face of constant environmental and cultural pressures that push for fragmentation, particularly in postmodern cultures (McAdams, 1996). This religion-as-integration hypothesis appears to be a promising one that is in need of further empirical scrutiny. If there are inherent integrating tendencies within persons (Ryan, 1995), might not these be spiritual in nature?

In his careful analysis of stories of men and addiction, Singer (1997) found that a key ingredient that distinguished between those men who relapsed and those who maintained sobriety was the ability to fit their personal life narrative into a larger, transcendent story. Singer employs the term "embeddedness" to describe this location of personal identity in "an inherent state of connectedness" in which boundaries between the self and otherness dissolve (p. 291). A greater recognition of embeddedness increased the likelihood that the men would be interested in making a generative contribution to society, by increasing their sense of obligation and responsibility and transcending their long-standing self-centeredness.

CONCLUSIONS

Divided consciousness appears to be part and parcel of the human condition. Conflict is also paradoxical. On the one hand, it is potentially destructive. It leads to poor physical and mental health, interferes with healthy communication in relationships, and disrupts performance and problem-solving on a variety of tasks. Conflict prevents a person from effectively regulating goal-directed action. Without the direction and coherence supplied by a dominant integrative pattern, life seems fragmented or aimless. Optimal psychic health and well-being occur when different elements of personality are integrated into a more-or-less coherent whole. On the other hand, conflict is also required for personal growth, and has been empirically linked with creativity (Sheldon, 1995).

Csikszentmihalyi (1993) has argued persuasively that humanity's fate rests on the establishment of "the complex self"—differentiated (individual uniqueness) and integrated (active concern for the well-being of others). To direct evolution, we must first transform the self. Similarly, Kovac (1996) has contended that "the progressive evolution of mankind depends predominantly on the primary transformation of man" (p. 193). Spirituality, in its essential nature, is concerned with personal transformation. "Integration is the direction in which evolution must progress to secure us a liveable future," writes Csikszentmihalyi (1993, p. 157). There may be no greater need than for integration of the self, which is of greater significance than the desire for personal happiness and well-being. Personal spiritual transformation may be a surer road to wholeness than other strategies that have been attempted and that have failed.

CHAPTER SEVEN

Personal Goals and Life Meaning

When author and theologian C. S. Lewis (1970) was asked which of the world's religions gives to its followers the greatest happiness, he replied "While it lasts, the religion of worshipping oneself is the best" (p. 33). He explained that he did not turn to religion to make him happy: He always knew that a bottle of port wine would do that. Although much of the scientific literature on subjective well-being may lead one to a different conclusion, there is more to living a good life than being happy. For instance, there is a difference between a meaningful life and a happy life. In some cases the two may be correlated, but in others they may not be. Some researchers have called for a broader definition of well-being than what has commonly been adopted in the literature, convinced that systematic investigation of concepts such as wisdom, meaning, and purpose in life should supplement the widely adopted measures of happiness and life satisfaction (Ryff & Singer, 1998). The previous chapter examined the role of spiritual goals in fostering personality unification and integration. As we saw, integration can occur quite independently of whether a person is satisfied or happy with his or her life, yet it is a crucial part of an overall sense of well-being.

This chapter is concerned with the examination of "personal meaning" as an empirical and theoretical construct. As ultimate concern is often centered around existential issues, it is time to address the meaning construct and see how it might enable us to better understand linkages between spirituality, motivation, and personality.

Personal goals provide a basis for evaluating hedonically based models of well-being and meaning-based conceptions. At this point we need to confront the relation between these two conceptions and what the implication is for understanding the good life. Empirically, meaning and happiness are relatively independent components of well-being that are often associated with different predictors. For example, some research shows that having children predicts meaning in life but not happiness (Baumeister, 1991). Meaningfulness appears to be a necessary yet insufficient condition for long-term happiness. A meaningful life is one that is characterized by a deep sense of purpose, a sense of inner conviction, and assurance that in spite of one's current plight, life has significance. Whereas it is possible for a life to be imbued with significance yet devoid of happiness, (e.g., the lives of some religious martyrs), it is impossible for long-term happiness to occur in a life devoid of meaning. Although meaningfulness may not guarantee high levels of positive emotional well-being, an absence of meaning and purpose portends unhappiness. A meaningful life will be a life filled with rich and varied emotions, both pleasant and unpleasant. The philosopher Robert Nozick (1989) persuasively demonstrates this conception in the following quote:

> It is not clear that we want these moments [of happiness] constantly or want lives to consist wholly and only of them. We want to experience other feelings too, ones with valuable aspects that happiness does not possess as strongly . . . we want experiences, fitting ones, of profound connection with others, of deep understanding of natural phenomena, of love, of being profoundly moved by music or tragedy . . . experiences very different from the bounce and rosiness of the happy moments. What we want, in short, is a life and a self that happiness is a fitting response to—and then give it that response. (p. 117)

Variables that provide both a sense of meaning and purpose as well as enjoyment and pleasure should be especially strong predictors of overall well-being. Relationships are one example. Most people find their interpersonal relationships both deeply meaningful and a prime source of positive emotions. Goals have consistently predicted well-being outcomes because different characteristics of them are associated with both enjoyment and meaning. For example, B. R. Little (1989) found that high-level, abstract projects were associated with greater meaningfulness whereas low-level, more short-term projects were linked to greater immediate enjoyment (the meaningfulness vs. manageability trade-off). Religion may exert its powerful influence on well-being through this dual process as well, serving not only as a framework for meaning but also as a deep and lasting source of joy and hope (Myers, 1992).

There is perhaps no more powerful example of the need to bring together both psychological and theological perspectives than in the study of how people cope with the inevitable adversities and suffering of life.

Psychological trauma "leads us into the realm of the unthinkable and fundamental questions of belief" (Herman, 1992, p. 7). Dealing with personal trauma requires a person to become a philosopher, therapist, and theologian.

MEANING AND GROWTH THROUGH SUFFERING

> Consider it pure joy whenever you face trials of many kinds, because you know that the testing of your faith produces perseverance. Perseverance must finish its work so that you may be mature and complete, not lacking anything.
> —JAMES 1:2–4, *NIV*

The presence of suffering in people's lives poses a challenge for theories of subjective well-being. That suffering is endemic to the human condition is an inescapable conclusion that derives from centuries of philosophical, theological, and psychological literatures. One of the basic truths that forms the cornerstone of virtually all of the world's great wisdom traditions is that life is suffering. For example, the first of the Four Noble Truths of Gautama Buddha is that life inevitably involves *dukkha* (suffering). At the same time, the psychological literature on subjective well-being has concluded that "most people are happy" (Diener & Diener, 1996). In survey research, most people, around the world, whether living in advantaged or disadvantaged circumstances, report a positive level of well-being. How can most people be happy given the ubiquitousness of suffering, pain, and adversity? Is it possible for this apparent paradox to be resolved? Perhaps people are masterful self-deceivers who fool themselves into thinking they are happy when they are really miserable. On the other hand, perhaps they are masterfully adaptive creatures who able to transform adverse circumstances into opportunities for personal growth, lasting happiness, and quality of life even in the face of pain and suffering. Most of the world's great religious traditions embrace suffering in the name of spiritual growth, as the quote from James's epistle at the outset of this chapter reveals. While the self-deception hypothesis cannot be totally ruled out, it is this second alternative that will be defended in this chapter. Evidence will be reviewed demonstrating that life is often elevated to the sublime precisely under those conditions that might be expected to produce the most pain and misery. The purpose of this chapter is to review the current state of psychological knowledge regarding adjustment to extreme life circumstances. In particular, the literature on the construction of life meaning following adversity will be presented and synthesized. The following questions will be addressed: What are the sources of human suffering?

What are the psychological and interpersonal consequences of suffering? What are the responses to suffering? How are people able to derive meaning from traumatic circumstances? What elements are involved in the reconstruction of meaning? Specifically, the chapter will focus on the concept of "stress-induced growth," the general term for positive well-being that appears to occur not only in spite of suffering and adversity, but perhaps even because of such trials. Paradoxically, it may be that deep and lasting well-being requires a modicum of suffering. Understanding how suffering can eventually result in heightened sensitivity to life's pleasures, and the role that personal goals play in coping, are the major purposes of this chapter.

THE NATURE OF SUFFERING

The nature of human suffering—its sources and the human response to it—have been preeminent concerns throughout the history of humankind. Although the problem of suffering is traditionally considered to fall within the purview of theology, psychological and theological forces recently have joined together in an attempt to unravel the mysteries of suffering. Many excellent modern treatises on suffering have been written from a psychotheological perspective (e.g. Anders, 1994; Fichter, 1981; Peters, 1994; Pruett, 1987; Taylor & Watson, 1989; Tedeschi & Calhoun, 1995; Vash, 1994). Clark (1958), in his classic psychology of religion text, distinguished two primary loci of suffering: external and internal origins. External sources include both natural catastrophes as well as atrocities suffered at the hands of others. Internal suffering is that which is brought about by a person's own actions. These internal sources include temperament, neurosis, conflict, and separation from God, according to Clark. A contemporary expansion of Clark's taxonomy might include addiction and other self-defeating traits, and disease-prone characteristics such as hostility and self-centeredness. Tedeschi and Calhoun (1995) compare and contrast religious and psychological perspectives on suffering. One of the more thorough modern treatments of suffering was contributed by ethicist David Little (1989), who delineated four categories of "legitimate suffering": retributive suffering, therapeutic suffering, pedagogical suffering, and vicarious suffering. He viewed these as a critical minimum to classify experiences and events as producing suffering. Both therapeutic (psychological growth) and pedagogical (becoming wiser as a consequence) suffering are germane to this chapter. Little points out that one of the purposes of religion is to provide a meaningful account of why people suffer. For the purpose of this chapter, it is also important to distinguish between the experience of pain and the experience of suffering. Some individuals are born without the capacity to feel physical pain and thus undergo considerable suffering in their lives due to this rare condition. Then there are those unusual persons who actually enjoy physical pain. The focus of this chapter will not be on physical pain, but rather on psychic pain that occurs in response to extreme life circumstances, and the positive changes that appear to be potentiated by this psychic pain.

It would not be an exaggeration to say that the current period in history could be depicted as the "age of trauma." The use of trauma and suffering language is often stretched to refer to nearly any unpleasant event, no matter how slight in severity ("I suffered through my pastor's sermon," "I just broke up with my boyfriend of 2 weeks and it was *so* traumatic"). Not long ago I was walking down the hallway near my office and I overheard a student confiding in her friend, "I'm turning 22 on Sunday and I feel *so* old." This chapter will focus not on these "garden-variety" traumas, but instead on massive upheavals that have the capacity to produce changes in every realm of a person's life. Psychologists cannot scientifically address the why of human suffering; that is usually left up to the theologians, philosophers and even anthropologists like Geertz (1966), who noted that the problem of suffering is "an experiential challenge in whose face the meaningfulness of a particular pattern of life threatens to dissolve into a chaos of thingless names and nameless things" (p. 46). Psychologists specialize in studying the human response to suffering. In the context of well-being, psychologists can and have examined the personal and social resources that enable a person to transcend tragedy, to grow, and to experience gains in the face of significant loss. After a review of the literature on positive outcomes of suffering, the second part of this chapter reviews the concept of meaning as it applies to suffering and well-being and personal goals.

STRESS-INDUCED GROWTH

The possibility that life's adversities may serve as a catalyst for personal growth is a familiar theme in psychological, philosophical, and theological writings. Sapolsky's (1994) tongue-in-cheek analysis of the commonplace nature of these reports depicts stress-induced growth as "the trendiest subject in the field" (p. 250). In his study of self-actualizers, Maslow (1955) noted that "the most important learning experiences . . . were tragedies, deaths, and trauma . . . which forced change in the life-outlook of the person and consequently in everything that he did" (p. 23). Until recently, the psychological evidence for the general proposition that losses may lead to gains has been limited mostly to anecdotal reports using global measures of perceived growth. Recently, significant strides have been made as researchers have begun to empirically assess the degree of personal growth in the aftermath of severe life stressors. These efforts have included the development of theoretical models designed to account for the processes by which traumas can lead to benefits (Aldwin, 1994; Antonovsky, 1987; Schaefer & Moos, 1992; Tedeschi & Calhoun, 1995; Vash, 1994), empirical investigations of the relations between various forms of traumatic experiences and subsequent reported positive life changes (Folkman & Stein, 1997), and the design of self-report questionnaires to measure individual differences in perceived positive life changes following personal crises (Park, Cohen, & Murch, 1996; Tedeschi & Calhoun, 1995).

Schaefer and Moos (1992) formulated a conceptual framework designed to account for the processes by which positive outcomes of life crises occur. They postulated three major types of positive outcomes: enhanced social resources (primarily deeper, more satisfying relationships), enhanced personal resources (becoming more self-reliant, positive changes in values and goals), and enhanced coping skills, including emotion regulation. Schaefer and Moos identify several specific crises that can generate these positive outcomes, including divorce, bereavement, and chronic or terminal illness. Finally, they specify four sets of factors that affect the likelihood that positive changes will in fact follow these significant life crises: event-related factors, personal factors, environmental factors, and coping resources. Event-related factors include characteristics of the stressor such as its controllability, its duration, and its expectedness. Personal resources include temperament, prior exposure to crises, and resiliency factors such as dispositional optimism, hardiness, self-control and self reliance, and a sense of coherence (Antonovsky, 1987). Environmental factors pertain primarily to adequacy of social support and community resources.

The theoretical framework offered by Schaefer and Moos served as the basis for Park et al.'s (1996) study of stress-related growth in college students. These authors developed the Stress-Related Growth Scale (SRGS), a 50-item inventory designed to assess perceived positive changes in personal resources, social relationships, and coping skills. Operating from a standpoint of stress-initiated growth, items are phrased in terms of what the person learned as a result of confrontation with a significant stressful life event (e.g., "I learned to accept myself," "I learned to be nicer to others," "I learned to ask others for help"). Park et al. report that the scale is unidimensional and possesses both high internal consistency as well as test–retest reliability. In terms of validity, scores on the scale are significantly associated with reports of growth by significant others and are uncorrelated with social desirability. In a prospective study, the SRGS predicted increases in optimism, social support, and positive affect over a 6-month period. Significant predictors of stress-related growth included the initial stressfulness of the event (greater stressfulness predicting more growth), intrinsic religiousness, and the coping strategies of positive reinterpretation and acceptance.

Tedeschi and Calhoun (1995) have formulated a model of personal transformation following suffering, and have been engaged in a series of studies to test their model. They describe three broad categories of perceived benefits that arise from the struggle with adversity: self-confidence, enhanced personal relationships, and changed philosophy of life. These bear close resemblance to the three categories of benefits described by Schaefer and Moos (1992). Tedeschi and Calhoun then present a self-regulation model to account for the process of growth following trauma: It begins with changes in higher-order schemas regarding the nature of reality, followed by a positive evaluation of the self and the world in terms of meaningfulness, manageability, and comprehensibility. Central to their formulation is the intriguing notion that positive changes occur in the person as a result of the struggle with trauma, and "perhaps only because of the trauma" (p. 87).

Tedeschi and Calhoun (1995) developed the Post-Traumatic Growth Inventory (PTGI), a 21-item questionnaire wherein respondents are asked to indicate the degree to which various benefits have occurred subsequent to experiencing a traumatic life event. The scale factors into five components, which the authors labeled New Possibilities, Relating to Others, Personal Strength, Appreciation of Life, and Spiritual Change. The scale possesses satisfactory test–retest and internal reliability, and is uncorrelated with social desirability. Females scored higher on all factors except for New Possibilities. Scores on the PTGI are modestly positively correlated with the five factors of personality: extraversion, openness to experience, agreeableness, and conscientiousness (r's ranging from .29 to .16). Scores on the PTGI were also shown to distinguish between those who had experienced a severe trauma and those who had not, with the severely traumatized scoring higher on the overall scale and on all factors compared to those who had experienced less severe trauma.

Methodological Issues in Stress-Induced Growth Research

Like other research using mental health outcomes, the research on stress-induced growth is beset by the following criterion problem: How do we know that self-reports of growth are to be taken at face value? To what degree are reports of positive changes following crises real versus illusory? Self-reports of subjective well-being appear to contain substantial amounts of validity (Diener, 1995). Yet there are additional complications in the measurement of stress-induced growth research. One concerns the operation of demand characteristics for people who have experienced major crises. Given the widespread use of positive illusions (Taylor & Brown, 1988) to manage affect combined with the prevalence of strong normative beliefs concerning stress-induced growth ("If it doesn't kill me, it makes me stronger"), people may feel pressured to acknowledge the benefits of their struggles whether or not any objective benefit has actually accrued. Another argument against the validity of self-reports of growth is that trauma often induces denial and other defenses that prevent the full impact of the event from registering. However, this argument is weakened by the fact that denial is most likely to be an initial reaction to the event, while stress-related growth measures are typically taken well after this initial reaction to the crisis. Yet another problem stems from temperament influences on well-being, which are typically not assessed and therefore not controlled for in these studies. Happiness returns to a set-point rapidly after even major events (Suh, Diener, & Fujita, 1996), so people may use the covariation between unpleasant events and subsequent positive emotion as an indication of stress-induced growth. Corroboration of self-report through knowledgeable others (Park et al., 1996) is one solution to this problem. Outcome measures of growth and other positive changes need to be sensitive to detecting even minor benefits that might elude a global appraisal. The research on positive growth following trauma is still in its infancy, and future efforts will surely include more sophisticated assessment of the many facets of growth. A recent volume expertly reviews the many challenges that confront researchers intent on understanding how people might benefit from life's adversities (Tedeschi, Park, & Calhoun, 1998).

GROWTH AS MEANING MAKING

The rapidly accumulating literature on stress-induced growth places considerable importance on the concept of "meaning" as a key theoretical construct mediating between stress and positive change. Meaning is often defined in terms of having experienced positive changes or perceived benefits as the result of the event. Growth is possible to the degree to which a person creates or finds meaning in suffering, pain, and adversity. Interest in the subject of personal meaning has increased dramatically in recent years. While philosophers have cooled to the topic of meaning in life, social scientists have been warming to it and are gradually recognizing that despite its vague and boundless nature, the topic can be seriously and fruitfully investigated (Ryff, 1989; Wong & Fry,

1998). The scientific and clinical relevance of the personal meaning construct has been demonstrated in the personal well-being literature, in which indicators of meaningfulness predict psychological well-being, while indicators of meaninglessness are regularly associated with psychological distress and pathology. Originally arising within an existentialist perspective, contemporary psychological research has shown that *meaning matters*. The conclusions that a person reaches regarding matters of ultimate concern—the nature of life and death, and the meaning of suffering and pain—have profound implications for individual well-being. The meaning construct has been used as an outcome measure in well-being research as well as a proximal predictor of well-being (see Park & Folkman, 1997, for a comprehensive review). Meaning is conceptualized in most research as a relatively independent component of well-being, and researchers have recently advocated including it in conceptual models of well-being, quality of life, and personal growth (Compton et al., 1996; Ryff & Singer, 1998). Recent empirical research has demonstrated that a strong sense of meaning is associated with life satisfaction, while a lack of meaning is predictive of depression (Reker & Wong, 1988; Wong & Fry, 1998). The literature on meaning is enormous; thus, no attempt will be made to extensively cover or synthesize it here (see Wong & Fry, 1998, for a review). Rather, in this next section of the chapter, I will review selected studies on changes in meaning in the aftermath of adversity.

There is a vast area of research dealing with the personal meaning that is derived from various adverse life circumstances, including illness, disability, divorce, and other serious personal losses. Perhaps the classic study on meaning in the face of adversity was conducted by Taylor (1983), in her study of women with advanced breast cancer. She distinguished two forms of meaning: meaning-making attributions regarding the perceived cause(s) of the cancer and future-related meanings pertaining to implications of the disease for their future lives. A variety of attributions were provided to explain why these women believed they had contracted cancer, but, interestingly, no specific attributions predicted adjustment any better than any other attributions. It appeared that it was the ability to find *any* meaning that was crucial. In their study of incest survivors, Silver, Boon, & Stones (1983) came to a similar conclusion. The ability to find *any* meaning in the experience was associated with better social, emotional, and occupational adjustment, whereas those women who continued to search for meaning but whose search had come up empty experienced psychological distress and ruminative thoughts concerning their experiences that continued, in some cases, for 20 or more years after termination of the incest. At least some were able to find positives in their plight. One woman responded, "I learned over the years that nothing as bad as what I had been through was going to happen again. Now I know there is virtually nothing I cannot overcome" (p. 90).

Schwartzberg (1993) studied how HIV-positive gay men make sense of AIDS. Using an interview format with 19 HIV-infected men, Schwartzberg explored the strategies these men used to make sense out of their plight. Meaning was established in a variety of ways, and their responses were organized by Schwartzberg into 10 categories: HIV as catalyst for personal growth (74%), HIV as belonging (74%), HIV as irreparable loss (74%), HIV as punishment (68%), HIV as a contamination of one's self (58%), HIV as a strategy for personal gain (47%), HIV as a catalyst for spiritual growth (42%), HIV as isolation (37%), HIV as confirmation of one's powerlessness (32%), and HIV as relief (21%). These 10 responses were then collapsed into four overall frameworks, which were labeled (1) high meaning, (2) defensive meaning, (3) shattered meaning, and (4) irrelevant meaning. Of these, the most common pattern was high meaning, in which "subjects were able to transform this information from despair to challenge, from psychological disequilibrium to catalyst for growth, to a reinvigorated appreciation of life" (p. 486). Consistent with the stress-induced growth literature, several of the men viewed their infection as a condition to be valued, that presented for them the opportunity to uncover previously dormant wisdom or inner strength. While these initial findings are intriguing and indicate the potential of life-affirming consequences of adversity, there is as yet little data on how these differential meanings relate to either subjective well-being or to objective outcomes such as mortality or survival time.

Also concerned with HIV, but from the perspective of caregiving, is the research of Folkman and her colleagues (Folkman & Stein, 1997; Stein et al., 1997), who have been engaged in series of studies examining how the caregivers of AIDS patients or HIV-infected men cope with the challenges and demands of their unique situation. They have focused on depressed mood in caregivers following bereavement. A key variable explaining adjustment appears to be finding positive meaning in caregiving. Those caregivers who viewed their caregiving experience as a deeply meaningful one exhibited lower levels of depression following the loss of their partner. Positive meaning in this situation was derived from multiple sources, including the knowledge that one had provided valuable support and reduced the suffering of a significant other to the degree it was possible.

Two other studies offer examples of the positive role of meaning-making in coping with bereavement. Edmonds and Hooker (1992) examined perceived changes in life meaning following the death of a family member. Grief was negatively associated with scores on the Purpose in Life test, a widely used measure of overall meaning in life. A finding suggesting the presence of stress-induced growth was that the majority of individuals (71%) reported a positive change in life goals as a result of bereavement. McIntosh et al. (1993) found that religious beliefs were used to construct meaning for parents who had lost a child to Sudden Infant Death Syndrome. Those parents who had found meaning within a religious framework had significantly less distress 18 months postloss as well as greater positive well-being. Both positive well-being and distress were measured separately in this study, and, interestingly, meaning through religion was associated more strongly with positive well-being than it was with the alleviation of distress. This is somewhat surprising in that religion is often turned to for the reduction of pain in the face of inexplicable suffering; indeed, some have taken the extreme position that suffering "is the basic reason for religion" (D. Little, 1989, p. 53). It would appear that when life is viewed from an eternal perspective, suffering in the here-and-now takes on a circumscribed, temporary meaning and is therefore more manageable. A religious or spiritual worldview provides an overall orientation to life that lends a framework for interpreting life's challenges and provides a rationale for accepting the challenges posed by suffering, death, tragedy, and injustice (McIntosh et al., 1993).

Personal Goals and Meaning

Among the elements in a person's meaning system that are used to construct meaning in the face of adversity, personal goals have recently been highlighted (Emmons, Colby, & Kaiser, 1998; Folkman & Stein, 1997). Goals appear to be prime constituents of the meaning-making process. As motivational constructs, goals are an important source of personal meaning and provide structure, unity, and purpose to people's lives (Baumeister, 1991; McAdams, 1993; Reker & Wong, 1988). Reker and Wong identified three levels of personal meaning: cognitive, affective, and motivational. The motivational component includes values and goals that provide guidelines for living (Reker & Wong, 1988), orienting a person to that which is valuable, meaningful, and purposeful. Goals play a major role in two forms of coping that will be described shortly. Goals are also attractive units for understanding meaning making in a methodological sense, given the existence of psychometrically sound personal goal assessment methods that were described in Chapter 2.

Although little hard data yet exist on the subject, theorists from various perspectives have shown widespread agreement that adversity contains the potential for reorganizing and refocusing a person's goals, values, and priorities. Traumatic events precipitate meaning crises, raising questions pertaining to the purpose and meaning of one's life and the nature of suffering and justice in the world, as the person struggles to answer both why the event occurred and what the implications will now be for one's future. Goals are used to construct meaning; finding or creating meaning in the face of suffering often involves changing or revising one's fundamental goals, concerns, and values. Case histories and other anecdotal evidence point to shifting goal priorities in the face of extreme life events (the prototypical example being an increase in "communal" goals following diagnosis of a life-threatening disease). Vash (1994) takes the position that adversity serves as a "wake-up" call that causes people to focus inward and evaluate their lives, including a reexamination of priorities and goals. This reprioritization has been postulated as a common response to affliction in cancer patients (Taylor, 1983), individuals with AIDS or those who are HIV-positive (Folkman & Stein, 1997), heart attack victims (Affleck, Tennen, Croog, & Levine, 1987), and persons with physical disabilities such as spinal cord injuries (Vash, 1994) and neuromuscular disorders (Keany & Glueckauf, 1993). In a goals framework, adaptation to loss requires relinquishing untenable goals, generating new goals, and developing pathways for their attainment that enable the restoration of meaning and purpose in life. Freund and Baltes (1998) refer to these processes as selection, optimization, and compensation.

Folkman and Stein's Model

Recently, Folkman and Stein (1997) have developed a model of stress and coping that places preeminence on goal processes. Their theory originates within a goal-theoretical perspective of emotion in which affective states are seen as a function of the status and nature of one's goal strivings. Whether affect is examined in terms of discrete short-term states (emotions) or, as described in Chapter 3, long-term individual difference characteristics (subjective well-being), there is widespread agreement that goals and related constructs such as concerns and commitments play an essential role in determining the quality and intensity of affective experience (Frijda, 1986; Klinger, 1977; Lazarus, 1991; Oatley, 1992; Ortony, Clore, & Collins, 1988). These various goal theories of emotion postulate that discrete emotional states are the results of goal-relevant appraisals (Lazarus, 1991; Oatley, 1992). Affect plays a role in determining one's commitment to goals, affect energizes goal-directed behavior, and affect serves as feedback informing a person of the status of his or her goals.

Folkman and Stein (1997) go beyond this rudimentary formulation and present a theory of coping specifying the conditions under which various forms of coping lead to adaptive or maladaptive outcomes. Specifically, their intent is to understand how goals are involved in the maintenance of positive emotions under deteriorating life circumstances. Successful coping requires the dual process of recognizing and disengaging from unrealistic and unattainable goals, and the ability to generate new goals that are personally meaningful, realistic, and attainable. To maintain or to recover well-being in the face of adversity, people must be flexible goal-strivers, recognizing when to continue to strive and when to eliminate or revise goals. Folkman and Stein (1997) developed a method for analyzing goal processes in narratives produced by the caregivers of men with AIDS. Caregivers' ability to engage in goal-related activities and events that they found positive and meaningful was a strong prospective predictor of positive psychological states a year following their partner's death. Spiritual and religious goals and beliefs were among those that most strongly helped participants cope with caregiving and bereavement. Their work is notable as it explores the process of goal setting and goal revision in sustaining well-being under difficult circumstances.

Goals may be especially important components of the meaning-making process because they are involved with different coping processes. Pargament (1996) distinguished between two forms of coping: conservational and transformational. Conservational coping refers to the preservation of that which is personally meaningful in the face of threat or loss, while transformational coping refers to the development or acquisition of new sources of meaningfulness after the immediate threat has passed. These two forms of coping exist in a dialectical relation to each other over time and are processes that "guide and sustain the person throughout the life span" (Pargament, 1996, p. 217). Personal goals are likely to be involved in both forms of coping, as the person first seeks to maintain coherence in the face of threat by increased commitment and renewed striving to certain goals and then gradually by reexamination of priorities and goals. Brandstadter and Renner (1990) made a similar distinction between tenacious goal pursuit and flexible goal pursuit, and found that while both styles were related to subjective well-being, flexible goal pursuit attenuated the negative impact of unsuccessful goal attainment on life satisfaction.

As mentioned previously, data on the relation between goals and adjustment in the face of adversity is difficult to come by. The Edmonds and Hooker (1992) study cited earlier asked subjects to indicate if their goals in life were changing as a result of bereavement, and if so, in what ways. The majority of individuals (71%) reported a positive change in life goals. A more extensive attempt to study the role of personal goals in coping with loss was conducted by Emmons, Colby, and Kaiser (1998).

We examined the link between personal goal systems and reactions to personal losses in two studies involving both college student and community adult samples. We anticipated that goals would be used to derive meaning following trauma: Recovery from loss should be partially a function of the development of and investment in new goal pursuits. Relatedly, we sought to determine whether commitment to specific types of goals (e.g., intimacy, personal growth, spiritual) promote the acceptance of and adaptation to loss. A related question was whether goal conservation or goal transformation was more likely following loss. Narrative accounts of loss and probing questions regarding life-goal change revealed that goal change is not a necessary consequence of traumatic loss. While the majority of participants did report change of some sort with respect to their goals, 40% did not. Changes in striving intensity—enhanced commitment, focus, and purpose—appear to be more common than changes in goal setting (i.e., content). Goal conservation appears to be nearly as common a response to trauma as goal transformation. Second, the results of our studies indicated that a lack of goal change, and not goal reformulation, is associated with recovery from experiences of loss. Perhaps the need for continuity during major life transitions fosters both goal conservation and facilitates adaptation to the stressor. Stressful life experiences were also associated with both negative and positive appraisals of one's goals. That is, people who reported more difficult life events were more ambivalent about their goals, rated them as more difficult to attain, and tended to strive for extrinsic reasons. Interestingly, however, these individuals invested more value and appear to be more committed to their goals compared to persons with lower levels of life stress. This might be taken as a further example of stress-induced growth.

Persons who were more committed to intrinsically satisfying spiritual and religious goals were more likely to say that they had both recovered from the loss and found meaning in it. Recovery and finding meaning were associated with being committed to the goals of "pleasing God," "experiencing personal growth," and "engaging in religious traditions." People who rated extrinsic goals of "being popular," "looking young," and "being able to attract a sexual partner" as important were less likely to have found meaning in their loss and less likely to say they had recovered from it. When it comes trying to make sense out of a traumatic experience, the content of what a person is trying to do does matter. Not only that, the meaning-making process, and eventual recovery from the loss, is facilitated to the degree that the content of a person's goals contains a search for the sacred. This finding is in agreement with the extensive and burgeoning literature demonstrating the effectiveness of religion in coping with life stress (e.g., Brown, 1994; McIntosh et al., 1993; Pargament, 1996; Park et al., 1996; Schumaker, 1992). In contrast, persons who were primarily preoccupied with self-focused goals were coping more poorly with the loss. The retrospective nature of this research precludes making strong inferences on the role of goals in the coping process. On the other hand, it would be foolhardy to assume that goals are irrelevant to coping with trauma. The goal construct has several advantages over dispositional and coping constructs for research on personality and illness (Elliot & Sheldon, 1998).

Self-transcendent spiritual goals—goals that connect the individual horizontally with others and vertically to a higher power—appear to facilitate the recovery process. In Chapter 5, I described a number of reasons why persons who commit themselves to spiritual goals experience more positive states of well-being. Perhaps the most central of these is that religion or spirituality can provide a unifying philosophy of life and serve as an integrating and stabilizing force that provides a framework for interpreting life's challenges and provides a resolution to such concerns as suffering, death, tragedy, and injustice. For many people, a religious meaning system and its associated goals may be the most reliable way to make sense out of pain and suffering. Taylor and Watson (1989) stated that "suffering stands at the very center of a religious response to the world" (p. 12). Religious beliefs and goals are powerful elements in personal meaning systems as they are relatively immune from disconfirmation (Tedeschi & Calhoun, 1995) and allow for conservational as well as transformational coping (Pargament, 1996). Once again, to quote Geertz (1966), "As a religious problem, the problem of suffering is, paradoxically, not how to avoid suffering but how to suffer, how to make of physical pain, personal loss, worldly defeat or the helpless contemplation of others' agony something bearable, supportable—something, as we say, sufferable" (p. 10). Future research needs to explore what types of religious goals are most effective in restoring meaning in the face of suffering, and the mechanisms by which these goals are effective. For instance, the richness of metaphor that religious systems provide (e.g., viewing major life changes as involving the death and burial of an old life and a resurrection to a new one) may be a potent means of deriving meaning from suffering (Crabtree, 1991; Rambo, 1993).

FUTURE DIRECTIONS:
GOALS AND PERSONAL GROWTH

Although the study by Emmons, Colby, and Kaiser (1998) did not provide definitive answers to how goals can aid in fostering stress-induced growth, it did demonstrate the potential that a goal-theoretical perspective can contribute to the understanding of adaptation following loss. Several changes in the characteristics of goal systems may have a positive impact on development. For example, it is possible that a reduction of conflict between goals and/or a change in goal content could lead to higher levels of functioning for individuals. Another avenue for growth includes an increase in goal complexity, or the variety of objectives a person is trying to accomplish. For example, the larger the variety of areas in which an individual has vested interests (i.e., work, family, leisure, etc.), perhaps the less likely that a loss in one area will completely devastate the person. Future studies aimed at understanding changes in goal content as a function of the experience of trauma may find it necessary to postulate a stage- related model of change. In particular, change is unlikely to involve a sudden all-or-none transformation; rather, a more gradual metamorphosis in one's purposes may be the norm. Following trauma, there is a powerful need to maintain the integrity of one's conceptual system (Epstein, 1991). As a result, a rapid reorganization of one's goals is both unlikely and ill advised. The need to develop new sources of self-validation through transformation in goal hierarchies must be balanced by maintaining the integrity of one's conceptual system. Indeed, the lack of goal change following a personal upheaval such as loss serves precisely this basic need for self-coherence and continuity. Goal continuity can have a stabilizing effect on the self during life-transitional periods. For example, it has been shown to promote psychosocial adjustment following retirement (Robbins, Lee, & Wan, 1994). Goal transformation might be associated with short-term distress since the process of relinquishing valuable previous commitments can be a wrenching one. Goal conservation, on the other hand, might be linked to short-term psychological benefits but to poorer outcomes in the long run, if the person is unable to move on to new goal pursuits.

In his analysis of the dynamics of religious conversion, Rambo (1993) makes a similar point that conversion is rarely dramatic. He outlines a three-stage process by which persons both develop the necessary orientation for change and consolidate change following initial conversion experiences. Separation, the first stage, involves the repudiation of previously held beliefs that are inconsistent with the new worldview. Transition, the second stage, is characterized by a reprioritization and transformation of beliefs. The third and final stage, consolidation, is marked by the acceptance and affirmation of the new belief system. Goal reformulation following trauma may follow a similar stage process. In this process, the individual must first disengage from or modify previously held goals prior to embracing new sources of meaning.

Breed and Emmons (1996) identified ways in which personal goals might be incorporated into grief management programs. They had 49 participants in a grief support group rate the extent to which they had discussed their respective current personal goals with their deceased partner, whether each goal was one they jointly pursued with that person, and the extent to which they believed the loved one would have supported the goal. Subjects who had discussed the goal with the loved one prior to his or her death and who had pursued other goals together scored lower on measures of psychological well-being and generally appraised their goals more negatively. Perhaps spouses were pursuing the goal out of a sense of obligation to their deceased partners. Recall that not all personal goals are, in fact, personal. Joint pursuit was negatively related to control and project initiation, which offers support for the conjecture that a sense of obligation was involved. Alternatively, perhaps the spouses lacked the skills or personal efficacy to successfully bring the project to completion. Individuals who expressed faith that their loved one would have supported their goal were better adjusted and appraised their goal more positively. Support was associated with perceived project importance, control, and value congruency.

The fundamental task facing the bereaved is that of relinquishing ties to the spouse while simultaneously maintaining an attachment (Shuchter & Zisook, 1993). Attachments are maintained through symbolic representations, rituals, and living legacies—extensions of the personality or other features of the deceased that are incorporated into his or her self-image. A commitment to personal goals or projects that the deceased person either was personally committed to or that the survivor believed would have been valued by the person appear to play an important role in the continuation of the relationship. At the same time, an enhanced attention to these goals should help the bereaved cope, transform the loss into an eventual gain, and help the survivor to feel as if the loved one's memory is being kept alive. A gradual transition from goals that were jointly pursued with the deceased to a reformulation of goals that would have been supported by the deceased loved one may, at least in the short-term, allow a reasonably adaptive solution to the dilemma of moving on while remaining connected.

MEANING, HAPPINESS, AND WISDOM: THE BIG THREE?

Nozick (1989) posed the question, "What is wisdom and why do philosophers love it so?" (p. 267). Given the recent surge of psychological interest in the topic (e.g., Aldwin, 1994; Baltes & Staudinger, 1993, Csikszentmihalyi, 1993; Kramer, 1990; Sternberg & Ruzgis, 1994), one could rightly rephrase the question to "Why do psychologists love it so?" It is hard to disentangle the concepts of meaning, happiness, and wisdom, and perhaps it would be wise not to attempt a scientific dissection of them at this late point in the chapter. Suffice to say that wisdom is a valuable resource for living the good life; it is intimately a part and parcel of each of the major topics discussed in this chapter—stress-induced growth, meaning making, and goal striving. The Old Testament writer of the Book of Proverbs phrased it simply: "Wisdom is supreme; therefore get wisdom" (Proverbs 4:7, *NIV*). It can be one of the primary outcomes of stress-induced growth (Aldwin, 1994; Tedeschi & Calhoun, 1995), a resource for the identification of valuable and significant goals (as well as the pathway for reaching those goals), and the knowledge of when to disengage from goal pursuit. Wisdom is "being able to see and appreciate the deepest significance of whatever occurs . . . appreciating the ramifications of each thing or event for the various dimensions of reality, knowing and understanding not merely the proximate goods but the ultimate ones, and seeing the world in this light" (Nozick, 1989, p. 276). The concept of wisdom has not yet made deep inroads in the literature on subjective well-being, perhaps because of a bias toward emotion as a primary indicator of well-being. As conceptual models continue to distinguish among components of positive well-being, the contribution of wisdom to the formula for happiness will eventually be recognized. The goals construct can serve as an important bridge between the psychology of wisdom and research on subjective well-being (Freund & Baltes, 1998).

Two recent empirical studies are relevant to the distinction between meaning and happiness. Rather than demonstrating a complete independence of these constructs, however, the data are suggestive of a moderate positive association. King and Napa (1998) studied folk conceptions "of the good life." They asked participants to judge the desirability and moral goodness of a person's life as a function of the amount of happiness, meaning in life, and financial success of the person. Both meaning and happiness determined the desirability of a life, with meaning accounting for slightly more variance. Both of these overwhelmed wealth; meaning had an effect size six times that of wealth, while happiness had an effect size five times that of wealth. King and Napa's study indicates that meaning and happiness jointly determine overall quality of life, or at least judgments of what the constitutes the "good life."

McGregor and Little (1998) also emphasized the distinction between meaning and happiness, equating the two with what they referred to as integrity and efficacy, respectively. Integrity refers to how consistent one's goals are with core aspects of the self, and efficacy refers to how successful one is at achieving the goals. McGregor and Little's usage of the term "integrity" is quite close to our discussion in the previous chapter on personality integration. In fact, their research creates a bridge between the concepts of integration and personal meaning. Drawing on an associative network perspective, the authors build a model in which hypothesized positive linkages between aspects of the self contribute to personal meaning, whereas negative or conflictual relationships between elements are hypothesized to contribute to a sense of meaninglessness. Evidence was found to support the hypothesized meaning/integrity and happiness/efficacy links, though the correlations were modest (.22 and .37, respectively). Happiness and meaning were moderately correlated with each other (*r* = .46). Both this study and King and Napa's (1998) suggest that, in general, meaning and happiness tend to co-occur, although the variables contain enough unique variance to enable them to correlate with different criterion variables.

CLINICAL IMPLICATIONS

As I did in Chapter 3, I would like to conclude this chapter by briefly considering some of the implications of research on goals and meaning for clinical contexts.

One implication of the research reviewed in this chapter involves the distinction between meaning and happiness made by health care professionals. The research of Folkman and her colleagues (Folkman & Stein, 1997; Stein et al., 1997) makes it clear that it is possible to derive meaning from mundane activities even in the face of a deteriorating situation such as caring for a person who cannot recover, and that meaning occurs in the context of the goals toward which a person is striving. Providing avenues for meaning and enabling the person to derive a sense of purpose and meaning is an important and valuable alternative when the gravity of a situation appears to preclude positive emotions. Wong (1998) has developed a meaning-centered counseling program that is especially designed to help clients extract positive meaning from otherwise debilitating life situations. The identification of valuable and meaningful strivings and projects achievable in daily life is a critical component in meaning-centered counseling. Enabling a client to live a life that is deeper and ultimately more fulfilling often entails a reorganization of striving commitments along with increasing sensitivity to opportunities for their realization. Similarly, Lapierre et al. (1997) suggest that it may be possible to redirect the content of an elderly person's chronic goals from those that provide less meaning and purpose to more meaningful pursuits in conjunction with a life review process.

A second important implication of the research reviewed in this chapter is that given the crucial role that spiritual goals and commitments appear to play in the restoration of meaning, and in the positive changes that follow struggles with adversity, therapists and other professionals need to be both keenly aware and appreciative of their clients' spiritual and religious orientations (Kelly, 1995; Shafranske, 1996).

There seems to be a growing sensitivity to and acceptance of religion in the lives of their clients on the part of clinicians and an attempt to harness the power of these belief systems for healing.

CONCLUSIONS

It is intriguing (and unfortunate) that the stress and coping literatures and the subjective well-being literature evolved independently of each other and have tended to go their separate ways. The stress and coping framework has historically focused on the amelioration of psychological distress, whereas the well-being field is more concerned with positive evaluations of one's life. Very few studies have explicitly addressed the connection between well-being and coping. With the recent flurry of activity directed toward understanding positive changes produced by stress, the fields may begin to more closely parallel each other. Aldwin (1994) reports that there have been over 10,000 studies on the negative effects of stress and comparatively few on stress-induced positive outcomes, an observation that is reminiscent of Myers and Diener's (1995) claim of a similar imbalance of ill-being to well-being studies. The goals concept may serve as an integrative unit for bridging these separate but interdependent research traditions.

The survey research literature on subjective well-being (Diener & Diener, 1996) indicates that most people are happy. It is also a fact that adversity and suffering are realities of life that comprehensive theories of subjective well-being cannot ignore. Quality-of-life specialists must be cognizant of the ways in which people attempt to extract growth-enhancing features from personal trials and to create and foster conditions under which the potential for positive outcomes is increased. While most people may indeed be happy, their struggles have left them not only with greater opportunity to experience a wider range of emotions, but in many cases with deep transformations in character. Paradoxically, it may be that enjoyment of life is not only possible in the face of suffering, but that suffering may be one road to deep and lasting happiness. The research on well-being reviewed in this chapter suggests that "the good life" is not one that is achieved through momentary pleasures or defensive illusions, but through meeting suffering head on and transforming it into opportunities for meaning, wisdom, and growth, with the ultimate objective being the development of the person into a fully-functioning mature being. On this formula for happiness, age-old wisdom and modern science are in agreement.

CHAPTER EIGHT

Spiritual Intelligence: Toward a Theory of Personality and Spirituality

*I*n the preceding chapters, I have tried to establish a case for including spirituality and religiousness in research and theory in the psychology of personality. I have tried to do this by relating these spheres of human functioning to goal motivation and subjective well-being, matters of central importance in contemporary personality psychology. My goal has been to understand long-term individual differences in affective and cognitive well-being as a function of a person's motivational life. In order to do this, I have found it necessary to invoke a conception of spirituality that is general enough to represent the diverse meanings that spirituality holds for people in today's culture, yet is amenable to rigorous empirical study. As I have argued in Part I of this book, personality can be characterized by patterns of personal strivings, the typical or characteristic goals that people try to accomplish in their everyday lives. We saw in Part II that as a basic category of human experience, spirituality is revealed through ultimate concerns that center on the sacred. When people orient their lives around the attainment of spiritual ends, they tend to experience their lives as worthwhile, unified, and meaningful.

In this final chapter, I place these elements of the approach I have been developing in the first seven chapters into a larger, more inclusive theoretical framework. Recent advances in social-cognitive approaches to personality make possible the location of both personal strivings and spirituality within a common framework, one that represents an alternative way of conceptualizing spirituality within personality functioning. I call this framework *spiritual intelligence*. In this last chapter, I consider the possibility that spirituality might be conceived of as a type of intelligence, and I argue that this framework has the potential both to integrate disparate research findings in the psychology of religion and spirituality and to generate new research yielding fresh insights into the spiritual basis of behavior. The advantages of thinking about spirituality as an intelligence and the role of spirituality in personality, as well as in human behavior more generally, will be addressed in this chapter.

The cognitive-motivational framework for personality described in this book views people as intentional, usually (but not always) rational beings who, in concert with their social worlds, are engaged in a constant effort to strive toward personally defined goals. These goals emerge as a function of internal propensities such as motive dispositions and basic needs in conjunction with situational affordances that shape their expression across situations and over time. Motivation in the form of goal directedness is a major component of the cognitive approach to personality, and motivation is a key aspect of personality, as it lends coherence and patterning to people's behavior. Motivational units such as goals, motives, and values form a hierarchical system of which various levels could be activated depending upon environmental stimuli. Moreover, goals can be activated and subsequently guide cognitive and behavioral processing outside conscious awareness of the person (Bargh & Gollwitzer, 1994). For instance, the striving to "Be more humble" can be removed from conscious control and still be activated by situational cues sensitizing the person to opportunities for humility quite outside of the person's awareness. The cognitive approach to personality thus accommodates unconscious motivation and points to how the unconscious can be the source of goals independent of conscious intents and plans. Undoubtedly, much of the conflict between strivings that was discussed in Chapter 4 can be explained through the override of conscious intentions through counterintentional unconscious goals.

PERSONALITY, INTELLIGENCE, AND ADAPTIVE FUNCTIONING

Cognitive-motivational approaches have opened the door for a reconceptualization of the role of intelligence in personality. A recent volume (Sternberg & Ruzgis, 1994), dedicated to the interface of intelligence and personality, contained contributions from a number of distinguished researchers in these respective fields. There are a number of important contributions that the study of intelligence can make in understanding personality processes.

Educational psychologist Martin Ford (1994) highlighted four basic questions that should be asked about human functioning: He called them the process question, the content question, the effectiveness question, and the developmental question. These four questions are at the heart of personality psychology, and two are directly the focus of this chapter. The content question addresses the "what," or the having side of personality: What is the substance or meaning of a person's thoughts, goals, and actions? I have attempted to answer this question through an examination of the content of personal goal strivings. The effectiveness question deals with how well the person is functioning according to some criteria of success in life: happiness, life satisfaction, personality integration, social virtue, and the like. Ford (1994) contends that intelligence is the most commonly employed construct used to address the effectiveness question. Intelligence, then, is defined as "the characteristic of a person's functioning associated with the attainment of relevant goals within some specified set of contexts and evaluative boundary conditions" (p. 203).

Other current conceptions of intelligence similarly equate it with adaptive problem solving behavior, where problem solving is defined with respect to practical goal attainment and some sort of positive developmental outcome. According to Sternberg (1990), the adaptiveness of intelligent behavior is viewed in light of whether it can function to meet the goals of the organism. Intelligence has been recently defined as "the level of skills and knowledge currently available for problem-solving" (Chiu, Hong, & Dweck, 1994, p. 106), as "the ability to attain goals in the face of obstacles by means of decisions based on rational rules" (Pinker, 1997, p. 62), and as "a set of abilities that permits an individual to solve problems or fashion products that are of consequence in a particular cultural setting" (Walters & Gardner, 1986, p. 164). Problem solving is inherently goal directed; identifying a goal, locating and pursuing appropriate routes to the goal, and organizing potentially competing goals so as to maximize joint attainment are problem solving skills needed for the effective negotiation of one's adaptive landscape. Goal setting creates a series of problems to be solved, as it requires the formulation of strategies and plans to pursue these goals in the face of external obstacles or internal obstacles such as frustration, depression, anxiety, and conflict with other pursuits. For example, to "Live a life that is pleasing to God" requires an identification of and a commitment to a lifestyle that is pleasing to God, an identification of and a commitment to avoid that which is displeasing to God, and the inner self-regulatory mechanisms to deal with frustrations, temptations, and setbacks that will inevitably occur in trying to live a responsible and accountable life of this type in an environment that may lack supports for such efforts.

The central theme behind these definitions of intelligence is an emphasis on adaptive problem solving. The issues of what constitutes adaptive functioning and what is required to function adaptively are important ones. Dweck (1990) specified a set of three criteria to distinguish adaptive from maladaptive functioning. First, an adaptive pattern should minimize the potential for goal conflict. As we saw in Chapter 4, competing goals compromise effective functioning and are a major source of psychological and physical stress. Adaptiveness implies the coordination of multiple goals in the service of higher-order principles. The second criterion of an adaptive pattern is that it should enhance the probability of goal attainment. Third, an adaptive pattern should allow a person to effectively utilize a maximum amount of available information. Spirituality fosters adaptive functioning as it meets these criteria. Spirituality is associated with greater overall personality integration. The study by Sacks (1979) on the effect of spiritual exercises on integration of the self-concept, cited in Chapter 6, supports the supposition that spirituality can enhance congruency of the self. Successful self-regulation requires the effective management of systemic goal conflict, a skill which seems to be facilitated by spiritual practices and spiritual strivings.

Ford (1994) listed four prerequisites for effective functioning: (1) motivation, which determines the content of goal-directed action; (2) skills, which produce the desired consequences of movement toward goals; (3) biological architecture, which supports the motivational and skill components; and (4) a supportive environment (or at least one that is nonhindering) that facilitates progress toward the goal. Intelligent behavior, then, requires "a motivated, skillful person whose biological and behavioral capabilities support relevant interactions with an environment that has the informational and material properties and resources needed to facilitate (or at least permit) goal attainment" (p. 203). Intelligence within specific domains is revealed by the following: breadth of knowledge, depth of knowledge, performance accomplishments, automaticity or ease of functioning, skilled performance under challenging conditions, generative flexibility, and speed of learning and developmental change. In an elegant analysis, Ford crosses each of these seven evaluative dimensions with goal content domains, yielding estimates of personal intelligence in domain-specific areas, such as family relations, academic achievement, artistic competence, and parenting. The important theoretical contributions of Dweck and Ford should be kept in mind when later considering how spirituality can be a form of intelligence.

The Theory of Multiple Intelligences

One of the most influential and widespread theories of intelligence today is Gardner's theory of multiple intelligences (MI; Gardner, 1993, 1995, 1996; Walters & Gardner, 1986). As described earlier, Gardner defines intelligence as a set of abilities that are used to solve problems and fashion products that are valuable within a particular cultural setting or community. He postulates a number of relatively autonomous intellectual capacities, seven in his original formulation and eight in a recent revision. They exist as potentials inherent in each person, yet vary genetically in terms of individual competencies and potential for development. The eight distinct intelligences are linguistic, logical-mathematical, spatial, musical, bodily-kinesthetic, interpersonal, intrapersonal and naturalist. Each intelligence is a system in itself, as distinct from a global, unified entity of generalized intelligence. He argues that these separate intelligences exist on the basis of their cultural significance and their correspondence to underlying neural structures. Gardner presents evidence for the existence of these separate "computational or information processing systems" and suggests that cultures differentially structure conditions so as to maximize the development of specific competencies in their members.

In order to determine what competencies and abilities qualify as an intelligence, Gardner (1993) laid out eight criteria for distinguishing an independent intelligence: (1) an identifiable core operation or set of operations, (2) an evolutionary history and evolutionary plausibility, (3) a characteristic pattern of development, (4) potential isolation by brain damage, (5) the existence of persons distinguished by the exceptional presence or absence of the ability, (6) susceptibility to encoding in a symbol system, (7) support from experimental psychological investigations, and (8) support from psychometric findings. Although the list of intelligences is negotiable, these eight criteria are not; in the MI framework, for a human capacity to be considered an intelligence, it must satisfy the majority of the criteria.

Should spirituality be considered part of the human intellectual repertoire? What would happen if Gardner's criteria for the existence of an intelligence were applied to spirituality? Intelligence is the ability to solve problems and create products that have consequence in a particular cultural setting. Using this definition as a starting point, a legitimate case can be made for spirituality as a set of related competencies and abilities that provide a reasonable fit to the eight criteria. One immediate problem arises: How is spirituality to be defined? The degree to which the concept is defined broadly or narrowly may influence whether applying the language of intelligence makes sense. My impression is that overly restrictive definitions of spirituality have led Gardner to a premature dismissal of the possibility of considering spirituality as a form of intelligence. Before we examine spiritual intelligence vis-à-vis Gardner's criteria, the nature of what constitutes spiritual intelligence needs to be fleshed out.

SPIRITUALITY AS INTELLIGENCE

As reviewed earlier in this book, the many meanings of spirituality and religiousness have become the focus of vigorous theoretical and empirical scrutiny in recent years. At the same time, emerging trends in the psychology of religion have yielded an impressive but as of yet unintegrated account of adaptive functioning, in which spiritual beliefs, commitments, and practices have been associated with a wide variety of criteria of success in living including physical health, psychological well-being, and marital satisfaction and stability. A concept that has the potential to unite these various literatures would be serving an important integrative function. Spiritual intelligence might be that concept.

Spirituality in the Theory of Multiple Intelligences

In his writings on multiple intelligences theory, Gardner has made it clear that spirituality is not one of the intelligences. The following quotation is taken from a 1996 article: "I cannot enumerate how often I have been said to posit a 'spiritual intelligence' though I have never done so, and have in fact explicitly rejected that possibility both orally and in writings" (p. 2) He did admit, however, in an article the previous year that whether it is appropriate to add spirituality to the list of intelligences deserves discussion and study in nonfringe psychological circles (Gardner, 1995). In his most recent statement on MI, Gardner (in press) acknowledged the possibility of an "existential or cosmic intelligence," of which the core is a concern with "ultimate issues," but he dissociates this type of intelligence from a broader conception of spirituality eliminating the sacred core of spirituality, and viewing instead existential intelligence as "a strand of the spiritual."

It is my contention that spirituality does indeed meet Gardner's criteria for intelligence. First, though, we need to consider exactly what spiritual intelligence is. It may be useful to think of spirituality as comprised of a set of specific abilities or capacities. Although scientific research on spirituality is in a nascent form, enough information is currently available to be able to speak of specific abilities and competencies. In keeping with the intelligence-based conception of personality outlined earlier, spirituality may be conceptualized in adaptive, cognitive-motivational terms, and, as such, underlies a variety of problem-solving skills relevant to everyday life situations. Spirituality is postulated to be an aspect of adaptive personality functioning as it increases the probability of goal attainment. Spiritual concerns influence the way in which people construe their world, pursue strivings, and regulate their behavior in day-to-day living. This pragmatic approach to spirituality offers a perspective on spirituality that can counter the mistaken belief that spiritual states of mind are somehow on another "plane of existence"—a state of being that is phenomenologically valid, but has little relevance for problem solving and goal attainment in concrete life situations.

Before continuing this line of reasoning, however, a yellow cautionary flag must be raised. I do not wish to be misunderstood on the following important point. Viewing spirituality as an intelligence does not imply that spirituality is *nothing more* than problem solving, or that individuals merely "use" their spirituality in the service of goal attainment. To make this erroneous inferential leap would be an example of committing the "nothing-but" fallacy (Paloutzian, 1996) which has led to much misunderstanding in the psychology of religion. If there is one truth that can thus far be derived from the scientific study of spirituality, it is this: Spirituality is an enormously rich and diverse construct that defies easy definition or simple measurement. My thesis in this chapter is simply this: The adaptive processing of spiritual information is a part of intelligence, and individual differences in the skills with which such processing occurs constitute core features of personality. Spirituality can serve as a source of information to individuals, and, as a function of interests and aptitudes, individuals become more or less skilled at processing this information. Even with this caveat in place, criticism will no doubt still be directed toward this attempt to connect spirituality with intelligence. My goal is not to be controversial, nor to strip spirituality of its "soul," but rather to offer a conceptual approach that might help integrate existing literatures and stimulate new research efforts.

What Is Spiritual Intelligence?

Spiritual intelligence consists of a number of abilities and competencies that are constituent of a person's knowledge base or expertise. Spiritual intelligence is a framework for identifying and organizing the skills and abilities needed for the adaptive use of spirituality. In the spirit of Mayer and Salovey (1997), who opened the door of intelligence to encompass affective and motivational information, I wish to open the door even wider to allow for spirituality as part and parcel of intelligence. I am in general agreement with Chiu, Hong, and Dweck's (1994) desire to understand adaptive functioning within a broad and integrative framework of the person that is centered on goals and the affective-motivational mechanisms utilized in their pursuit. The only caveat that I would add is that spirituality be included in the framework. An account of effective functioning that ignores spiritual skills and abilities is likely to be theoretically and practically impoverished. Spiritual information is part of a person's knowledge base that can lead to adaptive problem-solving behavior. Spiritual formation is precisely about building an expert knowledge base, in this case, of the divine. Through, for example, the study of sacred texts and the practice of spiritual exercises, depth and breadth of a spiritual knowledge base is developed and refined. Religions have been described as "systems of information" (Bowker, 1976; Hefner, 1993), providing individuals with resources that are essential for living a good life. As we saw in Chapter 5, spirituality is organized around high-level goals, generally the most adaptive level of goal organization for effective functioning (Carver & Scheier, 1998; Emmons, 1996; Vallacher & Wegner, 1985).

The Components of Spiritual Intelligence

Based upon a review of the empirical literature in the psychology of religion and spirituality, at least five defining, interrelated characteristics of spiritual intelligence can be identified. There is nothing sacred about these five (in the sense that there are five and only five). At a minimum, spiritually intelligent individuals are characterized by (1) the capacity for transcendence, (2) the ability to enter into heightened spiritual states of consciousness, (3) the ability to invest everyday activities, events, and relationships with a sense of the sacred or divine, (4) the ability to utilize spiritual resources to solve problems in living, and (5) the capacity to engage in virtuous behavior or to be virtuous (to show forgiveness, to express gratitude, to be humble, to display compassion). These components are shown in Table 8.1.

The first two core components of spiritual intelligence deal with the capacity of the person to engage in heightened or extraordinary forms of consciousness. Transcendence connotes a rising above or going beyond the ordinary limits of physicality. It may describe rising above our natural world to relate with a divine being, or it may refer to going beyond our physical state to effect a heightened awareness of ourselves (Slife, Hope, & Nebeker, 1997). Themes of transcendence figure prominently

TABLE 8.1. Core Components of Spiritual Intelligence

1. The capacity to transcend the physical and material
2. The ability to experience heightened states of consciousness
3. The ability to sanctify everyday experience
4. The ability to utilize spiritual resources to solve problems
5. The capacity to be virtuous

in definitions of spirituality. For example, Elkins (1988) stated that spirituality is "a way of being and experiencing that comes about through awareness of a transcendent dimension and that is characterized by certain identifiable values in regard to self, others, nature, life, and whatever one considers to be the Ultimate" (p. 11). Transcendence has been described as a fundamental capacity of persons that enables a person to sense a synchronicity to life and to develop a bond with humanity that cannot be severed, even by death (Piedmont, in press).

Mysticism is an awareness of an ultimate reality that takes the form of a sense of oneness or unity in which all boundaries disappear and objects are unified into a totality. Consider author Alix Kates Shulman's (1995) description of a mystical experience that occurred while she was on a New York City subway train:

> Suddenly the dull light in the car began to shine with exceptional lucidity until everything around me was glowing with an indescribable aura, and I saw in the row of motley passengers opposite the miraculous connection of all living beings. Not felt; saw. What began as a desultory thought grew to a vision, large and unifying, in which all the people in the car hurtling downtown together, like all the people on the planet hurtling together around the sun—our entire living cohort—formed one united family, indissolubly connected by the rare and mysterious accident of life. No matter what our countless superficial differences, we were equal, we were one, by virtue of simply being alive at this moment out of all of the possible moments stretching endlessly back and ahead. The vision filled me with an overwhelming love for the entire human race and a feeling that no matter how incomplete or damaged our lives, we were surpassingly lucky to be alive. (pp. 55–56)

Spiritually intelligent individuals are those who may be especially skilled in entering such mystical states of consciousness. Considerable empirical work has been conducted on mystical experience (see Hood, Spilka, Hunsberger, & Gorsuch, 1996, Chaps. 6–7, for a review). Newberg and d'Aquili (1998) describe the social significance of unitary spiritual experiences arising from ceremonial religious rituals as well as the physiological benefits from individual meditation.

Sanctification encapsulates the third component of spiritual intelligence. Recall from Chapter 5 that to sanctify means to set apart for a special purpose—for a holy or a godly purpose. The sanctification of relationships, work, and goals is associated with enhanced relational and psychological well-being. Faith, through the sanctification of goals, appears to facilitate goal attainment. Contemporary research (Mahoney et al., in press; Dollahite, 1998) is documenting that there are important consequences of this sanctification process. Viewing one's parenting

(Hawkins & Dollahite, 1997) and grandparenting (King & Elder, 1998) behaviors as sacred obligations is related to an increased involvement in and commitment to these relationships. Hawkins and Dollahite (1997) have proposed a conceptual ethic of fathering as "generative work," and have empirically documented the contribution that religious beliefs and values make to caring for the next generation. King and Elder (1998) reported that, after controlling for background variables, religiousness was a significant predictor of family involvement. Religious grandparents engaged in more activities with their grandchildren, had more frequent contact with them, and were more likely to care for them when sick than were nonreligious grandparents. Each of these lines of research illustrates the potential benefits of sanctification in the interpersonal domain. The language of intelligence enables sanctification to be viewed as expertise that people might bring to bear to solve problems and plan effective action. The research of Emmons, Cheung, and Tehrani (1998), described in Chapter 5, suggests that personal strivings in life can become spiritualized through a process of sanctification. Religious beliefs thus transform goals into sacred strivings. If people believe that God is involved in their lives, goal striving becomes a collaborative activity with a higher power.

The fourth characteristic, the ability to utilize spiritual resources to solve problems in living, encompasses religious and spiritual coping (Pargament, 1997). Pargament reviews a large literature documenting the effectiveness of spiritual and religious resources in the coping process. Problem solving is the sine qua non of effective coping, as effective coping entails the implementation of problem-solving skills. Lazarus and Folkman (1984) define problem solving as "the ability to search for information, analyze situations for the purpose of identifying the problem in order to generate alternative courses of action, weigh alternative courses of action, weigh alternatives with respect to desired or anticipated outcomes, and select and implement an appropriate plan of action" (p. 162). These are abilities that are required when prior goals are abandoned and new goals are adopted. Spiritual conversions can shape the reprioritization of goals (Paloutzian, Richardson, & Rambo, in press), and the ability to revise and reprioritize goals are indicators of intelligence (Haslam & Baron, 1994). Furthermore, intrinsically religious individuals are more likely to be effective at handling traumatically induced stress; they are more likely to find meaning in traumatic crises and are more likely to experience growth following trauma than are less religious persons (Park et al., 1996).

The fifth and final component of spiritual intelligence refers to the capacity to engage in virtuous behavior: to show forgiveness, to express gratitude, to be humble, to display compassion and wisdom. There is no pretense here that this list is exhaustive. These virtues are included under the rubric of spiritual intelligence because of the salience of these concepts in virtually all major religious traditions. Conceiving of these inner qualities as virtues implies that these are sources of human strength which enable people to function effectively in the world. Synonymous with character traits, virtues are acquired excellences that "come closer to defining what a person is than any other category of qualities" (Zagzebski, 1996). As theoretical constructs, they are tightly linked with strivings. Just as strivings are never fully or permanently attained, the pursuit of excellence or moral perfection is never fully realized. Rather, in the words of early church leader Gregory of Nyssa, it is discovered in "continual striving" (Danielou & Musurillo, 1961). The final goal, or ultimate concern of virtue, according to Gregory, is to become known by God and become his friend.

Of long-standing interest to moral philosophers (Zagzebski, 1996) and theologians (Schimmel, 1997), psychologists are beginning to turn their attention to the study of these human strengths (Baumeister & Exline, in press). Baumeister and Exline (in press) proposed that self-control is the core psychological trait underlying the majority of virtues, and is essential for success in virtually all life domains. Similarly, self-control failures lie at the heart of the seven deadly sins: gluttony, sloth, pride, anger, greed, lust, and envy. In a later section, I elaborate on the benefits of two virtues in particular, humility and gratitude.

Identifying the core components of spiritual intelligence is the starting point for a theory of spirituality-as-intelligence. Whether or not there are more or less than these five characteristics is open to debate. At this early stage of development, the study of spiritual intelligence can benefit from a broad conceptual approach. As more is learned about spirituality through scientific research, eventually we may be able to speak more definitively of specific spiritual abilities and competencies at those abilities. The degree to which each of the abilities is related to each other and the independence of spiritual intelligence from other forms of intelligence are among the issues that await future theoretical and empirical inquiry. In the meantime, it is my belief that each of these five are justifiable aspects of what I am calling spiritual intelligence. Postulating spirituality as a set of related abilities and competencies is the first step for qualifying it as a form of intelligence, but we have yet to see how it stacks up against the accepted criteria of MI theory.

Does Spirituality Fit Gardner's Criteria?

How do we know what constitutes an intelligence? Meeting the criteria that Gardner (1993) proposed requires marshaling neurological, developmental, evolutionary, and psychological evidence. Fortunately, supportive data from each of these sources is available. What follows is a brief illustration from some of these areas. As Gardner places considerable faith in biological underpinnings of intelligence, it is that level of analysis that I primarily focus on.

Biology has sometimes been seen as preempting spiritual accounts of human functioning. A growing consensus, however, emerging among scientists and theologians is a position of "nonreductive physicalism" (Brown, Murphy, & Malony, 1998) that may provide the most complete view of human nature. Nonreductive physicalism understands human beings as a physical organism whose complex functioning gives rise to higher human capacities such as emotion, morality, and spirituality. The biological basis of spirituality and religiousness can be examined at three levels of analysis: evolutionary biology, behavior genetics, and neural systems. Arguments for the evolutionary plausibility of religion have come from a number of different quarters—from biologists, psychologists, anthropologists, and theologians (Burhoe, 1981; Hood et al., 1996; Kirkpatrick, in press; McClennon, 1997; Pinker, 1997; Wilson, 1978). From a psychological perspective, evolutionary biology has been proposed as providing an integrative framework for religious beliefs, practices, and commitments (Kirkpatrick, in press). Kirkpatrick contends that the universal success of religious belief systems is due to the fact that religion taps into a broad array of psychological mechanisms that evolved via natural selection to solve a specific class of problems faced by our ancestors. Furthermore, these mechanisms exist at both the cultural level, expressed through corporate religion, and at the level of individual, in terms of personal religiousness or spirituality. Kirkpatrick discusses a variety of evolved mechanisms that underlie a variety of religious beliefs and behaviors, including attachment, coalition formation, social exchange, kin-based altruism, and mating.

Evidence for the heritability of religious attitudes suggests genetic influence (Kendler, Gardner, & Prescott, 1997; Waller, Kojetin, Bouchard, Lykken, & Tellegen, 1990). Whether or not the core elements of what I am calling spiritual intelligence have a significant genetic component remains to be determined. However, given preliminary data from the field of behavior genetics on the heritability of religiousness, it would be surprising if spiritual intelligence turned out to be unrelated to genetic factors. There may also be implications of such a genetic link for interpersonal problem solving. In the largest study on personality and divorce ever undertaken, Jockin, McGue, and Lykken (1996) found that out of eleven personality traits, traditionalism was the strongest negative predictor of divorce risk. Traditionalism correlates about .5 with measures of religious commitment (Lykken & Tellegen, 1996) and is also highly heritable (Tellegen et al., 1988). Jockin et al. suggest that personality acts as a conduit of genetic influence on divorce risk.

The heritability of aspects of religiousness points to the role of biology without revealing relevant neural mechanisms. The growing field of neuroscience is also contributing to an understanding of the biological basis of spirituality in a way that might elucidate neural substrates. Recall that Gardner believes that specific brain structures underlie different types of intelligences, and that a given intelligence should be isolatable by studying brain-damaged patients. Brain scientists have begun to investigate the neural bases of religious and spiritual experience, both in terms of neural substrates of religious experience and their alteration in brain dysfunctions (Ashbrook, 1993; Brown, 1998; Jeeves, 1997; Newberg & d'Aquili, 1998; Saver & Rabin, 1997). Neuroscientists are demonstrating that distinctive neurobiological systems (primarily in the limbic regions) exist for religious experience, particularly for the mystical experiences of oneness and unity (d'Aquili & Newberg, 1998; Newberg & d'Aquili, 1998). The discovery of these neurobiological mechanisms strengthens the case for spirituality as an intelligence.

Yet another of Gardner's criteria for the existence of an intelligence is support from psychometric findings. This might be the easiest evidence of all to demonstrate, given the widespread availability of inventories to measure spiritual and religious states. Scales for the measurement of spiritual experience continue to proliferate at an alarming rate; some researchers have even called for a moratorium on the construction of new measures (Gorsuch, 1984). Piedmont (in press) presents data suggesting that spirituality may represent a heretofore unacknowledged sixth major dimension of personality and has shown its relative independence from measures of personality traits.

Space does not permit an exhaustive evaluation of the scientific literature on spirituality with respect to Gardner's eight criteria. In addition to the biologically based criterion, on which spirituality appears to fare quite well, spirituality would also appear to meet at least three other criteria: a characteristic developmental history (Fowler, 1981; Levenson & Crumpler, 1996), the existence of spiritually exceptional individuals (the Catholic mystics St. Theresa of Avila, St. John of the Cross, and the Sufi master Ibn Al-'Arabi are three excellent examples), and susceptibility to encoding in a symbol system (Gardner, 1993, in press; Tillich, 1957). Even with the truncated review presented here, there would appear to be an overwhelming amount of evidence stacking up in favor of the thesis that spirituality is, in fact, an intelligence.

Ibn Al-'Arabi as an Exemplar of Spiritual Intelligence

If we examine individuals considered to be spiritually exceptional, we can see how well the concept of spiritual intelligence fits. Consider, for example, the 12th-century Sufi mystic Ibn Al-'Arabi (Nasr, 1964). Ibn Al-'Arabi was well known for his capacity for transcendence and his ability to enter into heightened spiritual states of consciousness, and is known to be among the most prolific of Islamic mystical writers, listing at least 250 titles. It is clear from his writings that they are not merely the result of long mental and intellectual deliberations, but are also drawn from mystical visions and experiences. Ibn Al-'Arabi acknowledged that much of what he wrote came to him in mystical visions, while asleep and as direct revelation from God.

While well known as a spiritual master and teacher, he was also quite capable of applying his spirituality to everyday life. At the early age of 20, he married and was employed as Secretary to the Governor of Seville, spending much of his life in the formal study of politics, religion, and science. A strong advocate of the necessity of law and formal doctrine for the good of the community, he strictly applied this in his advice to political leaders. Yet at an early age he astounded his teachers and many influential leaders in his country, for instance, the philosopher Averroes, with his insightful views of mystical transcendence and how to integrate spirituality within one's life.

Ibn Al-'Arabi devoted the majority of his life to the study of mystical doctrine and experience and remained quite humble, compassionate, and virtuous. Well known and sought after as a spiritual master, his report of a particular incident while teaching gives insight into his character. Ibn Al-'Arabi reported:

> Their respect for me prevented them from being relaxed, and they were all very correct and silent; so I sought a means of making them more relaxed saying to my host, "May I bring your attention to a composition of mine entitled *Guidance in Flouting the Usual Courtesies*, and expound a chapter from it to you?" He answered that he would very much like to hear it. I then pushed my foot into his lap and told him to massage it, whereupon they understood my meaning and behaved in a more relaxed manner. (Austin, 1980, pp. 5–6)

The Adaptiveness of Spiritual Intelligence: Humility and Gratitude as Examples

At the conclusion of his book on experiential intelligence, Epstein (1993) closes by invoking spirituality as a pathway to the higher reaches of the experiential mind:

> The beacon for the spiritual path is faith in some power or force that transcends ordinary human understanding. Such faith is the source of a

broad perspective and a feeling of connectedness with a greater whole than exists in one's immediate experience. . . . This deep spiritual identification which transcends rational calculation, enables people to take the long view and experience its ultimate consequences without effort . . . at this, its highest level of functioning, the experiential mind becomes not a betrayer of long-range interests and concern for others, but a means for their achievement. (p. 267)

Epstein voices faith in the adaptiveness of a transcendent, spiritual orientation to the world. What is the evidence for the adaptiveness of the spiritual abilities and competencies that comprise spiritual intelligence? There is growing evidence that spiritually oriented lifestyles tend to protect people from unintelligent behavior, as, for example, from engaging in personally and societally destructive ways (Paloutzian & Kirkpatrick, 1995). There are certainly counterexamples, such as the ascetics who engage in "holy anorexia" (Wulff, 1997). Two characteristics of spiritual intelligence, humility and gratitude, in particular appear to enable effective functioning but have not received as much attention as other aspects of spirituality.

Although humility is often equated in people's minds with low self-regard and tends to activate images of a stooped-shouldered, self-deprecating, weak-willed soul only too willing to yield to the wishes of others, in reality humility is the antithesis of this caricature. Humility is the realistic appraisal of one's strengths and weaknesses—neither overestimating nor underestimating them. To be humble is not to have a low opinion of oneself, it is to have an accurate opinion of oneself. It is the ability to keep one's talents and accomplishments in perspective (Richards, 1992), to have a sense of self-acceptance, an understanding of one's imperfections, and to be free from arrogance and low self-esteem (Clark, 1992). In most philosophical treatments, humility is considered a virtue—a desirable characteristic to cultivate. Some of the most powerful spiritual, political, and scientific leaders of all time were characterized by a sense of perspective about their goals and themselves, refusing to succumb to the temptation of self-aggrandizement.

Humility has been tied to a number of personal and interpersonal life outcomes. In the health field, research has reported that a lack of humility—or the excessive self-focus found in the trait of narcissism—is a risk factor for coronary heart disease (Scherwitz & Canick, 1988). Another study found that narcissism in ex-spouses was a strong predictor of continued conflict between them, with predictable destructive consequences for their children (Ehrenberg, Hunter, & Elterman, 1996). Earlier we saw that informational search is part and parcel of problem solving. Humility has been associated with better informational search abilities and problem-solving efficiency (Weiss & Knight, 1980), and with ratings of teaching effectiveness (Bridges, Ware, Brown, & Greenwood, 1971). In a survey reported in the *National Law Journal* ("Jurors Prefer Lawyers," 1993), humility was the characteristic that jurors most admired in lawyers (perhaps due to its relative infrequency). Humility is also strongly linked with morality. Humility was a criterion that Colby and Damon (1992) used for identifying moral excellence in their in-depth study of the effective lives of moral exemplars. Thus, humility appears to facilitate success in a wide range of life endeavors, and is an example of the adaptiveness of spiritual intelligence.

Despite its presumed value in most of the world's religions and philosophies, psychologists have largely ignored the study of gratitude. Gratitude is a profoundly interpersonal emotion or virtue as well as a skill or an ability. It is the capacity to feel the emotion of thankfulness on a regular and consistent basis, across situations and over time in contexts that are appropriate to its elicitation. Conversely, ingratitude is a vice. An ungrateful person, one who lacks the ability to feel and display gratitude, is one whom regularly responds to the beneficence of others with resentment, hostility, or indifference. It has been argued that the disposition to acknowledge indebtedness is a source of strength, and the striving to feel and exhibit gratitude a sign of human perfection (Roberts, 1991).

A study recently conducted in my laboratory (Emmons & Crumpler, in press) examined gratitude and thanksgiving in everyday life. For 10 weeks, undergraduate students enrolled in a health psychology class were asked to complete a weekly log of their emotions, physical symptoms, and health behaviors. The weekly log included two global judgments where participants were asked to evaluate their life as a whole during the past week and their expectations for the upcoming week. In addition to filling out the weekly report, subjects were randomly assigned to one of three conditions. One-third were asked to simply record up to five major events or circumstances that most affected them during the week, one-third were asked to write down five hassles or minor stressors that occurred in their life in the past week, and the final third were asked to write down five things in their lives that they were grateful for.

Results indicated significant differences between the three groups on the outcome measures. Relative to the hassles and events group, participants in the gratitude group felt better about their lives as a whole and were more optimistic regarding their expectations for the upcoming week. The thankful group reported fewer physical complaints overall than the hassles group and spent significantly more time exercising than did subjects in the other two groups.

The gratitude intervention appeared to have an interesting unintended side effect on another area of functioning within the participants' lives. At the beginning of the study, they were asked to write down six goals or projects that they intended to pursue over the next 2 months. They were instructed that these projects might involve various domains of their lives including academics, family, friends, leisure, health, and religion. Two months later, they evaluated the degree of progress they had made on each of these six pursuits. Specifically, they were asked to rate how successful they had been in pursuing their goals, noting how much progress they had made toward each of their goals and how satisfied they were in the amount of progress they had made. Participants who had been in the gratitude group reported having made more progress toward their goals, on average, than participants in the other two groups. This fascinating finding suggests that the benefits of an attitude of gratitude extend beyond the domain of mood and well-being to encompass more specific indicators of successful life functioning—the attainment of concrete goals in life. The study provides some empirical confirmation of the venerable sayings that "thanksgiving leads to having more to give thanks for," and that there are benefits to "counting one's blessings, one by one" (Templeton, 1997).

Is There an Optimal Level of Spiritual Intelligence?

Spiritual intelligence has been conceived of in this chapter as largely a positive construct. There are benefits to being spiritually intelligent, just as there are benefits to any form of intelligence. Yet can one have too much of a good thing? Is there a downside to being spiritually intelligent? Is there an optimal amount of spiritual intelligence? Or to phrase the question differently, does it makes sense to describe someone as "spiritually unintelligent?" These are intriguing and vital questions to ponder. That there is a dark side to the religious life is beyond question. The construct of spiritual intelligence may be able to shed light on the possible harmfulness of religious beliefs or spiritually oriented lifestyles. Although a full treatment of this complex issue is beyond the scope of the remainder of this book, a few observations can be made. First, it is evident that a person could overdevelop his or her spiritual intellect while ignoring other areas of functioning. There is a danger in becoming spiritual to the point that one is unable to act effectively in the world, for instance, being so heaven focused that one is of no worldly good. Wilson (1989) describes a tension between otherworldliness and thisworldliness that often exists for religiously oriented individuals. It is easy to find examples of spiritually exceptional individuals who had highly developed capacities for transcendence and mystical experience who lived a life of passive detachment from this world. Other-worldly concerns must be balanced by this-worldly concerns for optimal effective functioning in life. A spiritually intelligent person is one who has achieved a harmonious balance of "heavenly and earthly spirituality" (Wilson, 1989, p. 174).

Relatedly, problems in functioning might also stem from an imbalance in the development of the specific components, or with an exclusive concern with some components to the neglect of others. For example, there may be those individuals who have highly developed capacities for transcendence or mystical experiences, yet have not cultivated the interpersonal virtues to the same degree. Conversely, there may be disadvantages to being too forgiving, or too grateful, or too humble, or too self-controlled. Perhaps extremes in each of the components are maladaptive. It should be remembered, however, that spiritual intelligence is an amalgam of several interrelated components, where the package as a whole can overcome limitations associated with deficiencies or overdevelopment of specific components. Whether problems in functioning stem from overdevelopment of the spiritual intellect, its underdevelopment, or the misapplication of spiritual information, it is clear that spiritual intelligence may have a sinister side that should not be underestimated with the emphasis on adaptive functioning.

Advantages of Spirituality-as-Intelligence

Viewing spirituality as intelligence enlarges the concept of spirituality to encompass meanings not typically associated with it. Spiritual intelligence enhances the plausibility of a scientific spirituality by locating spirituality within an existing acceptable psychological framework, one that has proven to be extremely useful in understanding the common ground between personality and behavior. It allows spirituality to become anchored to rational approaches to the mind that emphasize goal attainment and problem solving (Haslam & Baron, 1994; Pinker, 1997). Moreover, the spiritual intelligence framework opens the door for new links to be forged with areas of psychology that have been slow to examine spiritual issues, including developmental, cognitive, and as I have argued throughout the second half of this book, much of personality psychology. Conversely, an anchoring of spirituality in the intelligence tradition might enable theology to deal with challenges that arise from cognitive science and other naturalistic frameworks that attempt to model human nature (Brand, 1997).

Thinking about spirituality as an intelligence can provide a much-needed antidote to anti-religious intellectualism (Marsden, 1997), in which religious worldviews are seen as irrational, emotional, and illogical, akin to superstitious thinking. Religion and intelligence are two concepts that are not often uttered in the same breath. When their relationship is considered, they are most typically seen as mutually exclusive: Religiousness and spirituality are dismissed as disruptive and hindering of intelligent, effective functioning. Too often, a false dichotomy is set up between two extreme caricatures—one can either be a rational, logical, analytical, and skeptical thinker or a muddle-headed, touchy-feely, gullible spiritualist. Arguing from a similar perspective in their theory of emotional intelligence, Mayer and Salovey (1997) begin with the premise that emotion and intelligence are often viewed as incompatible because the former is perceived as an "intrinsically irrational and disruptive force" (p. 9). Instead of forcing a choice between faith and reason, this way of thinking about spirituality recognizes that spiritual processing can contribute to effective cognitive functioning rather than precluding it.

The construct of spiritual intelligence enables spirituality to be viewed as a quality that is more or less developed in different people, and may be cultivated as a form of expertise (Dixon & Baltes, 1986). There are individual differences in each of the five capacities and in overall spiritual intelligence; some people will be more or less spiritually intelligent than others, and more or less spiritually intelligent in different ways. While all human beings possess the potential for spiritual intelligence, personality differences and socialization experiences will raise it for some and lower it for others.

Spiritual intelligence provides an integrative framework for understanding the salutary effects of religion on psychological, physical, and interpersonal outcomes. The benefits of a spiritually oriented lifestyle have been reviewed in this chapter. To remind the reader of one example, the ability to invest one's relationships with a sense of the sacred is related to enhanced commitment, which leads to better, longer-term intimate relationships. Shifting domains, personal religiousness is a predictor of adherence to health care regimens (Naguib, Geiser, & Comstock, 1968; O'Brien, 1982), and adherence is generally wise (see Karoly, 1993, for application of an intelligence framework to the study of medical adherence). As the adaptive use of spiritual information, spiritual intelligence can contribute to positive life outcomes such as emotional well-being, positive social functioning, and an enhanced overall quality of life, each of which appear to benefit from exercise of the spiritual intellect.

Finally, in defining and measuring spirituality/religiousness, it is all too easy to conceive of spiritual and religious variables as passive, static, trait-like entities. Spirituality and religiousness become something that a person has or possesses (e.g., beliefs), or behaviors that are engaged in (rituals). Alternatively, viewing spirituality as a set of skills, resources, capacities, or abilities enables spirituality to take on active, dynamic properties. Spirituality not only *is* something, it *does* something. As a dynamic property of persons, spiritual intelligence provides an interpretive context for addressing important concerns in daily life, and enables researchers to address the "doing" side of spirituality, as well as the "being side" (cf. Cantor, 1990).

Spiritual Intelligence and Other Spiritual Constructs

What is the difference between spirituality and spiritual intelligence? I have defined spiritual intelligence as the adaptive use of spiritual information to facilitate everyday problem solving and goal attainment. Spirituality is a broader, more encompassing construct that has as its focus a search for the sacred. It is a search for experience that is meaningful in and of itself. Intelligence is the implementation of a set of tools to arrive at a more productive, effective, happier, and ultimately more meaningful life; spirituality determines how "meaningful" is defined. Spiritual intelligence is thus a mechanism by which people can improve their overall quality of life. Spiritual intelligence is largely a positive, adaptive construct, whereas spirituality may be positive or negative depending upon how it is expressed in particular contexts. As suggested earlier, those same skills might be applied inappropriately, in a destructive manner.

Spiritual intelligence may also be contrasted with other positive spiritual constructs that have appeared in the psychology of religion literature, including spiritual well-being (Ellison, 1983) and spiritual maturity (Hall & Edwards, 1996; Malony, 1988). Spiritual well-being is primary affective in nature, and encompasses both religious and existential well-being. Although it is based on an assumption of a *need* for transcendence, different people may be more or less skilled at developing ways to satisfy this need. Hall and Edwards developed the Spiritual Assessment Inventory, a measure of spiritual maturity from a Judeo-Christian perspective. It is based on a theory of spiritual maturity grounded in relational anthropology and object relations theory, and assesses two principle components: an awareness of God in one's daily life and the quality of one's relationship with God. Similarly, Malony (1988) developed the Religious Status Inventory to assess optimal religious functioning, or spiritual maturity. This inventory is based on eight theological categories (e.g., acceptance of God's grace and love, being repentant and responsible, being ethical, experiencing fellowship) and basically assesses whether individuals' faith is a strength or weakness for them. Measures of spiritual maturity tend to be based on developmental stage perspectives. I would expect that spiritual intelligent individuals would be spiritually mature and that they would also tend to score high on spiritual well-being. The absence of a comprehensive assessment instrument to measure individual differences in spiritual intelligence precludes an empirical documentation of these assertions at this time.

Cultivating Spiritual Intelligence

Postulating spiritual competencies and abilities to be relatively independent human faculties opens to the door to the possibility that they can be cultivated in a manner analogous to other types of intelligences. Gardner (1993) argues that communities selectively identify particular competencies for development and elaboration. If spiritual intelligence does indeed confer individual and societal advantages, if the world would be a better place if people were more "spiritually intelligent," the desirability and feasibility of strategic efforts to augment it ought to be investigated. Rather than forcing spirituality or religion on people because it is good for them or society, edifying people as to how spiritual and religious skills might lead to success in life may prove to be a more effective and lasting route to spiritual transformation. Just as educational programs have been developed to raise emotional intelligence (Salovey & Sluyter, 1997), spiritual skills could similarly be acquired and cultivated. After all, the purpose of character education programs (Lickona, 1991) is to foster spiritual virtues and spiritual maturity so as to produce productive and socially responsible members of society. A spiritually intelligent character education program would go beyond the teaching of socioemotional skills to include the basic spiritual competencies and abilities described in this chapter. For example, Lickona (1991) discusses how humility is an essential component of good character. It is also one of the components of spiritual intelligence, and is predictive of a variety of positive life outcomes.

CONCLUSIONS

I have tried in this chapter to provide a language for describing the relationship between personality and spirituality. It is my belief that progress in understanding spiritual influences in people's lives requires the identification of higher-order organizing principles that can integrate existing research and lead to new discoveries. Science often advances when a model with demonstrated utility in one field is modified and applied within another. Perhaps spiritual intelligence is one such concept that can stimulate progress in understanding the effect of a "functional" spirituality in people's lives. Spiritual intelligence provides an elegant and powerful framework for the organization and synthesis of existing information and for the generation of new knowledge. It suggests new domains of intelligent action in the world. The adaptive use of spiritual information is a significant aspect of what it means to be an intelligent, rational, and purposive human being, yet spirituality has not been studied as a component of theories of intelligence. Psychologists continue to divide and subdivide intelligence in many ways, but absent from such partitioning is a spiritual or religious way of knowing (Watts & Williams, 1988). Conversely, the potential explanatory and integrative force that intelligence can provide has been neglected by psychologists interested in religious and spiritual issues. An intelligence-based conception of spirituality can stimulate progress in the psychology of religion and can be determinative of future theoretical and research agendas. Hood et al. (1996) encourage researchers to examine constructs that originally derived their meaning from within religious traditions in order to "enliven the psychology of religion" (p. 198). Spiritual intelligence may be one such enlivening construct. It will likely profit from continued conceptualization, research, and debate in scientific circles.

SOME FINAL THOUGHTS

Looking Back

In a single volume, how does one do justice to the profound topics of motivation, spirituality, and personality on their own, let alone in their interaction? Humbly, and with much gratitude toward those who have blazed trails before me, I acknowledge that I have barely scratched the surface. I have described the research that has occupied my professional life for the past dozen or so years. My overriding goal in this book has been to build a model of how motivation and spirituality might come together in the person and what the implications of this interaction might be for how personality relates to important life outcomes. I have attempted to articulate and defend why a spiritual strategy is desirable for contemporary personality theory and research. My hope is that the research presented in this volume has not merely served as an academic discourse. For those who are uncertain how to proceed in their lives, the information presented in this book offers some guidelines for a psychology of spiritual possibilities of what makes life meaningful, valuable, and purposeful.

Looking Ahead

We are embarking on a significant period in the scientific study of spirituality. For personality and goal researchers, this means that we will be able to continue to move toward an understanding of the ultimate goals of human existence. There is reason to believe that the coming years will provide a period of unlimited opportunity and potential for pursuing truth through a blending of experimentation and revelation. The goals approach to spirituality shows that we need not compromise scientific rigor and precision in order to make progress in understanding what people find valuable, purposeful, and meaningful. On the contrary, rigorous methodology and precise conceptualization applied to issues of fundamental human concern will enable the continued growth of a sound infrastructure that will serve to generate new knowledge and its application. The biggest threat to understanding human personality is not the complexity of the subject matter, though that is considerable. The biggest threat to understanding is the failure to take seriously those phenomena which make us most human.

APPENDIX A

Personal Striving Assessment Packet

PART 1. STRIVING LISTS

One way to describe someone's personality is to consider the purposes or goals that the person seems to be seeking in his or her everyday behavior. We are interested in the things that you typically or characteristically are trying to do. We might call these objectives "strivings." Here are some examples of strivings:

Trying to be physically attractive to others
Trying to persuade others that one is right
Trying to help others in need of help
Trying to seek new and exciting experiences
Trying to avoid being noticed by others
Trying to avoid feeling inferior to others

Note that these strivings are phrased in terms of what a person is "trying" to do, regardless of whether the person is actually successful. For example, a person might be "Trying to get others to like me" without necessarily being successful.

These strivings may be fairly broad, such as "Trying to make others happy" or more specific, as "Trying to make my partner happy." Also note that the strivings can be either positive or negative. That is, they may be about something you typically try to obtain or keep, or things that you typically try to avoid or prevent. For example, you might typically try to obtain attention from others, or you might typically try to avoid calling attention to yourself.

You can see that this way of describing yourself is different from using trait adjectives (friendly, intelligent, honest). We do not want you to use trait adjec-

181

tives. Since you may have never thought of yourself in this way before, think carefully about what we are asking you to do before you write anything down.

We want you to provide us with a list of your strivings. Please write down at least 15 strivings in the spaces provided below. You may list additional strivings if you wish. Please keep your attention focused on yourself. Do not mentally compare the things that you typically do with what other people do. Think of yourself and your purposes alone. Be as honest and as objective as possible. Do not give simply socially desirable strivings or strivings which you think you "ought" to have.

You might find it useful to think about your goals in different domains of your life: *work and school, home and family, social relationships,* and *leisure/ recreation.* Think about all of your desires, goals, wants, and hopes in these different areas.

Take your time with this task; spend some time thinking about your goals before you begin. When you have finished, move on to Part 2 (Striving Assessment Scales).

I typically try to _____

I typically try to _____

I typically try to _____

I typically try to _____

I typically try to _____

I typically try to _____

I typically try to _____

I typically try to _____

I typically try to _____

I typically try to _____

I typically try to _____

I typically try to _____

I typically try to _____

I typically try to _____

I typically try to _____

I typically try to _____

I typically try to _____

I typically try to _____

PART 2. STRIVING ASSESSMENT SCALES

In Part 1, you listed a number of your personal strivings (things that you are "typically trying to accomplish"). In this task, we want you to make some ratings about each goal on your list. Begin by writing in your strivings in the left-hand column of the answer sheet (see top of p. 189). There is room for you to write in 15 strivings You will need to select the 15 that you believe best describe what you are typically or characteristically trying to do.

1. Happiness

How much joy or happiness do you or will you feel when you are successful in your striving? For example, suppose your striving is "Trying to stay caught up in studies." You would imagine how happy you would be if you were successful in keeping up with your studies and then pick a number from the scale below to express this degree of happiness. Write that number in the column marked "Happiness" on the answer sheet.

```
0 ———— 1 ———— 2 ———— 3 ———— 4 ———— 5
no happiness   slight      moderate    much       very much   extreme
   at all      happiness   happiness   happiness  happiness   happiness
```

2. Unhappiness

How much sorrow or unhappiness do you or will you feel when you fail to succeed in your striving? In this step, imagine that your are not successful in your striving. For example, suppose your striving is "Trying to control my anger." You would imagine how unhappy you would be if you failed to control your anger. Pick a number from the scale below to express this degree of unhappiness and write that number in the column marked "Unhappiness" on the answer sheet. It might be helpful to think of unsuccessful past experiences.

```
0 ———— 1 ———— 2 ———— 3 ———— 4 ———— 5
no unhappiness  slight       moderate     much         very much    extreme
   at all       unhappiness  unhappiness  unhappiness  unhappiness  unhappiness
```

3. Ambivalence

Sometimes, even when we are successful in reaching a goal, we are unhappy. Even success sometimes has its cost. For example, if you are "Trying to become more intimate with someone," and you succeed, you might also feel concern about being more tied down, having more responsibility, and being unable to date others, etc., despite also being pleased with the outcome. Choose a number from the scale below that indicates how ambivalent or unhappy you would be about succeeding at the striving and write that number in the column marked "Ambivalence" on the answer sheet.

0 ——————— 1 ——————— 2 ——————— 3 ——————— 4 ——————— 5
no unhappiness   slight   moderate   much   very much   extreme
   at all   unhappiness   unhappiness   unhappiness   unhappiness   unhappiness

4. Importance

Now we would like to know how important each of your strivings is to you in your life, or how committed you are to working toward each of your strivings. For example, if your striving is "Trying to get along with my family," you would choose a number from the scale below indicating how important it is to you that you get along with your family. If your striving is "Trying to avoid gossiping about others," how important is it that you don't gossip about others? Perhaps it is not very important, at least relative to your other strivings. Write that number in the column labeled "Importance" on the answer sheet.

0 ——————— 1 ——————— 2 ——————— 3 ——————— 4 ——————— 5
not at all   slightly   somewhat   moderately   very   extremely
important   important   important   important   important   important

5. Past Attainment

In your estimation, in the recent past (within the last month or so), how successful have you been in your strivings? We want you to estimate as best as you can the degree to which you have achieved success in each of your personal strivings. For example, if your striving is "Trying to stick to my diet" you would estimate how successful you had been in the past month at sticking to the diet. For this response, pick a number from the scale below and write it in the column marked "Attainment" on the answer sheet.

0 —— 1 —— 2 —— 3 —— 4 —— 5 —— 6 —— 7 —— 8 —— 9
0–9% 10–19% 20–29% 30–39% 40–49% 50–59% 60–69% 70–79% 80–89% 90–100%

6. Probability of Success

Next, we want you to estimate the overall likelihood that you will be successful in the future in each of your strivings. How likely is it (or how much do you expect) that you will succeed in your strivings? Think in terms of specific goals. For example, if one of your strivings is "Trying to lose weight," how likely is it that you will lose, say, 10 pounds in the future? Using the scale below, choose a number that corresponds to your best estimate of your chances in succeeding in the striving. Write that number in the column marked "Success" on the answer sheet.

0 —— 1 —— 2 —— 3 —— 4 —— 5 —— 6 —— 7 —— 8 —— 9
0–9% 10–19% 20–29% 30–39% 40–49% 50–59% 60–69% 70–79% 80–89% 90–100%

7. Environmental Opportunity

In this step, we want you to indicate how much life circumstances permit you to be successful in the striving. These circumstances can include your living situation, available resources, other people, etc. In other words, how much do circumstances around you typically help or hinder your attempts. For example, suppose your striving is "Trying to get enough exercise to stay in shape," but because of your schedule you can't find enough time to exercise. In this case, circumstances in your life would be hindering your striving. Choose a number from the scale below which corresponds to the opportunity typically provided you to be successful in the striving, then write that number in the column labeled "Opportunity" on the answer sheet.

Circumstances make it:

0	1	2	3	4	5
very easy	somewhat easy	neither help nor hinder	somewhat difficult	moderately difficult	very difficult

8. Effort

How much effort and energy do you generally expend in trying to be successful in the striving? Each of your strivings involves a different set of contributions from you—some take a lot of time, others may cost money, some inconvenience you, others drain you emotionally, etc. What we are interested in here is how much effort or energy it takes on your part to be successful in each of your strivings. Indicate this by using a number from the scale below, then write that number in the column marked "Effort" on the answer sheet.

0	1	2	3	4	5
requires no effort at all	requires very little effort	requires some effort	requires moderate effort	requires much effort	requires very much effort

9. Difficulty

In general, how difficult is it for you to be successful in each of your strivings? Think about the obstacles which you encounter, how much demand each striving places on you, your opportunity to succeed, etc. Using the scale below, come up with a judgment of generally how difficult you find trying to succeed in the striving, and place that number in the column marked "Difficulty" on the answer sheet.

0	1	2	3	4	5
very easy	moderately easy	somewhat easy	somewhat difficult	moderately difficult	very difficult

10. Social Desirability

How socially desirable do you think each of your strivings is? That is, do you think that other people believe the striving is one that they themselves would like to be characterized as having? For example, you might perceive that "Trying to stay caught up in studies" is a socially desirable striving, whereas "Trying to party as much as possible" is not socially desirable. Note that we are emphasizing social and not personal desirability. Regardless of whether you think the striving is desirable, how do you perceive that other people would view the striving? Pick a number from the scale below to indicate this social desirability judgment, and write that number in the column marked "Desirability" on the answer sheet.

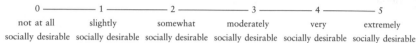

0	1	2	3	4	5
not at all	slightly	somewhat	moderately	very	extremely
socially desirable	socially desirable	socially desirable	socially desirable	socially desirable	socially desirable

11. Clarity

For each of your strivings, you may or may not have a well-formed idea or plan of how you will go about trying to be successful in your strivings. In this step, we want you to think about how clear an idea you have of what is required of you in order for you to be successful in the striving. For example, if your striving is "Trying to stay caught up in studies," you may have a clear idea of how much time you need to devote to each class, how much time to devote to nonacademic pursuits, etc. Alternatively, you may have little or no idea of how to go about staying caught up in your studies, perhaps simply because you haven't thought much about it. Use the scale below in making this clarity judgment, then write that number in the column marked "Clarity" on the answer sheet. What is required of me to accomplish my goals is:

0	1	2	3	4	5
very clear	quite clear	somewhat clear	somewhat unclear	quite unclear	very unclear

12. Progress

Consider how much progress you have been making toward your strivings. How satisfied are you with the amount of progress you have been making toward each of your strivings? Using the scale below, choose a number which best represents your satisfaction with how well you perceive yourself to be doing in each striving, then write that number in the column marked "Progress" on the answer sheet.

0	1	2	3	4	5	6	7
not at all satisfied			neutral				extremely satisfied
no progress or a setback							exceptional progress

13–16. Attribution

Past research suggests that people may be motivated to do something for many different reasons. In this task, we would like you to rate each of your strivings in terms of each of the following four reasons, using the following scale:

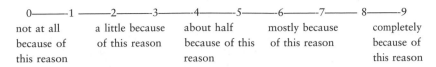

0——1 ——2——3——4——5——6——7——8——9

<table>
<tr><td>not at all
because of
this reason</td><td>a little because
of this reason</td><td>about half
because of this
reason</td><td>mostly because
of this reason</td><td>completely
because of
this reason</td></tr>
</table>

13. Extrinsic

You strive for this because somebody else wants you to or thinks you ought to, or because you'll get something from somebody if you do. Stated differently, you probably wouldn't strive for this if you didn't get some kind of reward, praise, or approval for it. For example, "Going to church regularly" might be a striving of yours because your parents would criticize you if you didn't go.

NOW: Please use the preceding scale to rate each of your 15 strivings on this reason, rating them in the same order that you wrote them into the grid. Use column 13 on the answer sheet, marked "Extrinsic."

14. Introjected

You strive for this mostly because you would feel ashamed, guilty, or anxious if you didn't. Rather than striving because someone else thinks that you ought to, you feel that you "ought" to strive for that something. For example, "Going to church regularly" might be a striving of yours because you would feel bad about yourself if you didn't go.

NOW: Please use the preceding scale to rate each of your 15 strivings, in the same order as before, on this reason. Use column 14 on the answer sheet, marked "Introjected."

15. Identified

You hold this striving because you really believe that it's an important goal to have. Although this goal may once have been taught to you by others, now you endorse it freely and value it wholeheartedly. For example, "Going to church regularly" might be a striving of yours because you generally feel this is the right thing to do.

NOW: Please use the preceding scale to rate each of your 15 strivings, in the same order as before, on this reason. Use column 15 on the answer sheet, marked "Identified."

16. Intrinsic

You strive purely because of the fun and enjoyment that striving provides. While there may be many good reasons for the striving, the primary "reason" is simply your interest in the experience itself. For example, "Going to church regularly" might be a striving of yours because the experience of being at church is genuinely interesting and enjoyable to you.

NOW: Please use the preceding scale to rate each of your 15 strivings, in the same order as before, on this reason. Use column 16 on the answer sheet, marked "Intrinsic."

17. Support

What impact do the important people in your life have on each striving? In general, what role do important others play in helping you achieve, or impeding (blocking or slowing down) the achievement of each striving?

For example, an important other may provide useful advice that aids you in achieving your striving(s). You may rate this impact as helpful if you feel the advice you received contributed to fulfilling the striving. Likewise, sometimes important others (either intentionally or unintentionally) hinder our progress toward certain strivings. For example, he or she may provide you with misleading advice or information on how to achieve a striving. In this case, you may want to rate the impact of this person as detrimental or impeding your progress toward your striving(s). There are even times when the same person can both help and hinder the progress toward personal goals. For example, a significant other may help you generate different ways to achieve a particular striving, but, at the same time, that person may make costly mistakes when trying to help you with your strivings and impede your progress.

For each striving, think about the person who has the most impact on that striving (either positive impact, negative impact, or both). Using a number from the scale below, rate the degree of support or hindrance that you usually receive from others for each striving:

1 = Extremely supportive of my efforts at achieving this striving
2 = Supportive of my efforts at achieving this striving
3 = Somewhat supportive of my efforts at achieving this striving
4 = Neither supportive of nor a hindrance to my efforts at achieving this striving
5 = Somewhat of a hindrance to my efforts at achieving this striving
6 = A hindrance to my efforts at achieving this striving
7 = An extreme hindrance to my efforts at achieving this striving

For each striving, write in the column under "Support" the number which corresponds to the role of the most important person related to each striving.

ID _____

STRIVINGS	Step 1 Happiness	Step 2 Unhappiness	Step 3 Ambivalence	Step 4 Importance	Step 5 Attainment	Step 6 Sucess	Step 7 Opportunity	Step 8 Effort	Step 9 Difficulty	Step 10 Desirability	Step 11 Clarity	Step 12 Progress	Step 13 Extrinsic	Step 14 Introjected	Step 15 Identified	Step 16 Intrinsic	Step 17 Support
1)																	
2)																	
3)																	
4)																	
5)																	
6)																	
7)																	
8)																	
9)																	
10)																	
11)																	
12)																	
13)																	
14)																	
15)																	

Striving Assessment Scales

PART 3. STRIVING INSTRUMENTALITY MATRIX (SIM)

This exercise is designed to have you think about how each of your personal strivings affects all of your other strivings. On the accompanying grid (see p. 190), you will note that there are 10 spaces across the top of the table and another 10 spaces on the left side of the table. Begin by writing 10 of your strivings in the spaces provided, along the top and left side of the grid. Since you may have provided more than 10 strivings, please select for this exercise 10 strivings only.

After you have finished writing your 10 strivings, start with the first striving at the top row of the table. Working vertically, compare your first striving with your second and ask yourself "Does being successful in this striving have a helpful or harmful effect (or no effect at all) on each of my other strivings?" For example, if your first striving is to "Do well in all of my classes" and your second striving is to "Spend time with my friends," you might see the first striving as having a harmful effect on the second, since if you are studying all of the time you won't have time to spend with your friends. It may be helpful to think of the ways in which you typically try to succeed in the striving. For example, if doing well in your classes entails studying with friends, then doing well has a helpful rather than a harmful effect on spending time with your friends. This is the way we want you to think about each pair of your strivings. For your response, there are 5 possibilities:

1. Succeeding in the striving has a *very helpful* effect on the other striving. In this case, put a "+2" in that space.
2. Succeeding in the striving has a *somewhat helpful* effect on the other striving. In this case, put a "+1" in that space.
3. Succeeding in the striving has **no effect** on the other striving. In this case, put a "0" in that space.
4. Succeeding in the striving has a *somewhat harmful* effect on the other striving. In this case, put a "–1" in that space.
5. Succeeding in the striving has a *very harmful* effect on the other striving. In this case, put a "–2" in the space.

Thus, the scale you will be using runs from –2 to +2. After you have finished comparing your first striving with the other 9, move on to the second striving and make the comparisons in the same manner. Then continue until the grid is completely filled out. Think about each comparison very carefully before you decide. If you have any questions, do not be afraid to ask.

ID _____

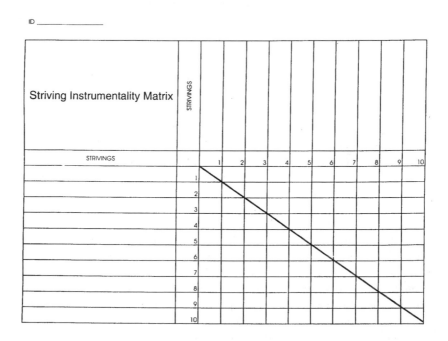

Personal Striving Coding Manual

GENERAL INSTRUCTIONS

Step 1 in the Personal Striving Assessment Packet (PSAP) asks respondents in an open-ended format to describe themselves in terms of the goals that they are characteristically trying to accomplish. This technique elicits an idiographic list of 15 personal strivings for each respondent. This manual describes 12 categories (approach vs. avoidance, intrapersonal vs. interpersonal, achievement, affiliation, intimacy, power, personal growth and health, self-presentation, self-sufficiency/independence, maladaptive/self-defeating, generativity, spiritual self-transcendence) that strivings can be classified into. In addition, the 15 strivings taken together can be rated for their level of abstractness–specificity (see Category 13). The categories are not intended to be exhaustive, rather, they are general categories that can be utilized for a variety of uses. Depending on the purposes of the research, other categories can be developed.

For each category, definitional criteria are given, followed by examples of strivings exemplifying that category. The categories are not mutually exclusive. All strivings can be coded in categories 1 and 2. However, a striving may not necessarily fit one or more of categories 3–12. If this should occur, it is better to leave these columns blank rather than force the striving into the category that "seems" best. A given striving can also overlap one or more motive categories (categories 3–6), but this is rare. For example, the striving "Forcing others to like me" would be scored for both affiliation and power.

RELIABILITIES

Intercoder reliabilities should be calculated. The appropriate statistic to assess agreement between coders on nominal scales is Cohen's kappa, which corrects for chance agreement. The formula for this statistic can be found in Fleiss, J. L. (1971). Measuring nominal scale agreement among many raters. *Psychological Bulletin, 76,* 378–382.

ADDITIONAL INFORMATION

To consult a published paper that employed the coding system, see Emmons, R. A., & McAdams, D. P. (1991). Personal strivings and motive dispositions: Exploring the links. *Personality and Social Psychology Bulletin, 17,* 648–654. An excellent source for coding narrative material in general is Smith, C. P. (Ed.). (1992). *Motivation and personality: Handbook of thematic content analysis.* New York: Cambridge University Press.

Category 1: Approach versus Avoidance

1. Does the striving refer to something positive or negative?
2. Does the person wish to approach, obtain, achieve, or keep the object of the striving, or does he or she wish to avoid, prevent, or get rid of the object of the striving?
3. Is the person trying "not to" do something? (Usually the words "avoid" "not" or "don't" will give it away.)

Examples of *avoidance* strivings (if not clearly avoidant, then code as approach):

"Not to feel bad when people dislike me for no known reason"
"Avoid escapism (fantasy and speculation about future)"
"Avoid letting anything upset me"
"Not to be possessive with my boyfriend"
"Not to feel inferior in social gatherings"
"Don't procrastinate"
"Restrain from arguing"
"Smoke less–drink less"
"Keep from wasting time"
"Be less self-centered"

Category 2: Intrapersonal versus Interpersonal

1. Does the striving refer to oneself or to others? Is there reference to the self or reference to others?
2. Is the striving *mainly* about oneself or *mainly* about others?
3. Is the object of the striving oneself or other people?

4. Does the striving refer to one's emotional state (intrapersonal) or the expression of emotion (interpersonal)?

Examples of intra- and interpersonal strivings:

"Try to help others" (inter-)
"Avoid worrying over financial setbacks" (intra-)
"Learn to deal with anger in a constructive way" (intra-)
"Please others" (inter-)
"Not to feel bad when people dislike me for no known reason" (intra-)
"Persuade others when I am right" (inter-)
"Be happier with my life" (intra-)
"Let people know I am angry with them" (inter-)
"Take care of myself" (intra-)
"Help others feel important"(inter-)

Category 3: Achievement

1. Reference to achieving or accomplishing a goal.
2. Competing with a standard of excellence.
3. Concern with competition, doing a task well, doing better than one has done before.
4. Reference to performance or winning.
5. Concern with success or accomplishment.
6. Trying hard to do something; expending effort.

Examples of strivings reflecting *achievement* concerns:

"Set high goals for myself and try to reach them"
"Realize my potential as far as a career is concerned"
"Achieve all that I can in as short a period as possible"
"Work toward higher athletic capabilities"
"Reach every career goal I set"
"Put my best effort into everything I do"
"Accomplish at least one main project a day"
"Use my time productively"
"Think about my future career goals"
"Save money"

Category 4: Affiliation

1. Concern for or desire to establish, maintain, or repair interpersonal relations.

2. Concern with seeking approval and acceptance from others.
3. Making efforts to win friends, an active striving toward friends.
4. Concern with preventing loneliness and rejection.
5. Concern with social acceptance and security in interpersonal relations.
6. Strivings that emphasize an active need to be with others, making friends, having others like the person.

Examples of strivings reflecting *affiliative* concerns:

"Maintain and improve relationship with my boyfriend"
"Be friendly with others so they will like me"
"Receive some form of physical affection"
"Meet new people through my present friends"
"Avoid being lonely"
"Be accepted in a social group"
"Keep in contact with long-distance friends so I won't lose them"
"Avoid being left out of conversations"
"Get enough attention and approval"
"Avoid confrontations with others"

Category 5: Intimacy

1. Commitment to and concern for another person.
2. Interpersonal relations involving positive affect: Love, friendship, happiness, peace, or tender behaviors.
3. Concern with experiencing a warm, close, and communicative exchange with another person.
4. Concern with loyalty and responsibility toward others.
5. Helping others; reciprocal communication and sharing.
6. Strivings that emphasize enjoying being with others, focusing more on the *quality* of relationships rather than *quantity*.

Examples of strivings reflecting *intimacy* concerns:

"Help my friends and let them know I care"
"Spend some time with my closest friends"
"Be a close, understanding friend"
"Help those who are less fortunate than myself"
"Accept others as they are"
"Have more patience with my girlfriend"
"Try to be a good listener"
"Give more than I expect to receive"

"Learn to express feelings of love toward my family"
"Be open about my positive feelings and be able to communicate them"

Category 6: Power

1. Concern about establishing, maintaining, or restoring power.
2. Concern with having impact, control, or influence over others.
3. Dominating, influencing, persuading, or convincing others.
4. Seeking fame or public attention (vs. success itself).
5. Concern for reputation or position.
6. Comparison and/or competition with others.
7. Influencing, controlling, or arousing emotions in others.
8. Giving help, assistance, or support when none is asked for.

Examples of strivings reflecting *power* concerns:

"Persuade others not to argue or fight with each other"
"Show that I am superior to others"
"Get others interested in my work"
"Force men to be intimate in relationships"
"Be the best when with a group of people"
"Be the dominant sibling in my family of six"
"Get other people to do the things I want to do"
"Dress in an unconventional style"
"Organize social gatherings and bring people closer together"
"Argue my point to the end"

Category 7: Personal Growth and Health

1. Improving, maintaining, or enhancing self-esteem.
2. Goals related to personal well-being, whether physical, emotional, mental, or spiritual.
3. Concern with being happier, or avoiding unhappiness, stress, anxiety, and other negative emotions.
4. Concern with improving or maintaining one's health; avoiding illness.
5. Concern with improving aspects of the self; characterological changes.

Examples of strivings reflecting *personal growth* and *health* concerns:

"Improve my health"
"Straighten out my values"
"Be more positive about myself"

"Be happier with my life"
"Develop a positive self-worth"
"Learn new skills and apply old ones"
"Avoid seeing the worst side of things"
"Avoid anxiety and other stressful emotions"
"Be strong while going through life's ups and downs"
"Mentally be aware of things around me"

Category 8: Self-Presentation

1. Concern with making a favorable impression on others.
2. Desiring to appear socially and/or physically attractive to others.
3. Concern with appearing intelligent, interesting, or desirable.
4. Concern with changing, maintaining, or improving one's image to others.
5. Concern with portraying a certain emotional state.

Examples of strivings reflecting *self-presentational* concerns:

"Appear intelligent to others"
"Avoid appearing outrageous"
"Make myself physically attractive"
"Impress others"
"Be concerned about my personal appearance at all times"
"Be self-confident in social situations when I am center stage"
"Be polite and well-mannered in the company of females"
"Act calm and cool when nervous"
"Always appear to be in a good mood"
"Try not to show negative emotions in public"

Category 9: Self-Sufficiency/Independence

1. Concern with being an individual, separated, autonomous from others.
2. Concern with seeking, establishing, or maintaining independence.
3. Avoiding being dependent or going along with the group.
4. Doing what one thinks is right.
5. Not having to depend on others.
6. Concern with asserting oneself.

Examples of strivings reflecting *self-sufficiency/independence* concerns:

"Do things without my friends every once in a while"
"Be myself and not do things to please others"

"Not be a pushover with others"
"Not be dependent on my boyfriend"
"Set time aside to get my thoughts together"
"Be an individual"
"Become financially independent from my parents"
"Not let other people take advantage of me"
"Stand up for myself and my beliefs"
"Not to depend on others to feel good about myself"

Category 10: Maladaptive/Self-Defeating

1. Strivings that reflect a lack of growth or adaptiveness.
2. A desire to avoid taking chances or accepting challenges that could result in positive growth or change.
3. Strivings that appear to be antithetical to those in Category 7 (Personal Growth and Health).

Examples of *maladaptive/self-defeating* strivings:

"Do as little as possible"
"Avoid things I'm not good at"
"Avoid calling attention to myself"
"Make everyone like me"
"Be perfect at everything"
"Do things that annoy others"
"Avoid voicing my opinion"
"Avoid the truth when faced with unpleasant facts"
"Avoid circumstances that I may fail in"
"Be accepting of everyone"

Category 11: Generativity

This category refers to strivings that relate to a goal of providing for the next generation, a desire for symbolic immortality, a desire to be needed by others, and belief in the fundamental goodness of human life and of the self. The expression of generativity in strivings can take the form of the following categories:

1. References to creating something, or having the desire to do so.
   Examples:
     "Be creative"
     "Find ways to make the most of my creative abilities"
     "Write and publish the book I've been thinking of for years"

2. Giving of one's self to others—tangible or intangible—or the desire to do so. Examples:

> "Contribute to my community"
> "Provide assistance to my elderly and ill mother"
> "Be involved with improving my community"

3. Reference to purposeful and positive interaction with the younger generation. Examples:

> "Help my kids with schoolwork"
> "Help my son play baseball"
> "Be a good father"
> "Be a good role model for my daughters"
> "See that my children get the best education possible"

4. Symbolic immortality: reference to leaving a legacy, having an enduring influence, or leaving behind products that will outlive one's physical existence. Examples:

> "Make a lasting contribution to my agency's mission"
> "Feel useful to society"
> "Make my life mean something"
> "Make a lasting contribution in my profession and avocation"

Category 12: Spiritual Self-Transcendence

Spirituality is the process by which persons affirm a nonmaterial reality that is beyond or is larger than themselves and attempt to align their lives with that reality. Spiritual, self-transcendent strivings thus refer to goals that are oriented above and beyond the self. They reflect a commitment to concerns that are larger than the individual. To transcend the self means to extend outward, toward others (horizontal transcendence) and/or to an ultimate reality (vertical transcendence). The expression of self-transcendence in strivings can take many forms, including but not limited to the following four dimensions:

1. **Divine awareness:** *Strivings that involve an acknowledgment of and a desire to relate to a higher power, or to gain knowledge of that higher power.*

> "Deepen my relationship with God"
> "Learn to tune into higher power throughout the day"
> "Appreciate God's creations"
> "Be filled with joy, peace, and happiness from knowing God"

2. **Universal equality:** *Strivings that reflect social responsibility and a sense of*

equity—*keeping promises, meeting obligations, conforming to social and moral rules, promoting fairness, justice, reciprocity, or equality, avoiding unfair or unjust actions.*

> "Treat others fairly"
> "Be more forgiving"
> "Defend those who have been treated poorly"
> "Deal with others with compassion and grace"

3. **Oneness/Unity:** *Strivings that reflect an integration of the individual with larger and more complex units: with other cultures, with humanity as a whole, with the natural landscape.*

> "Achieve union with the totality of existence"
> "Become one with the cosmos"
> "Immerse myself in nature and be a part of it"
> "Approach life with mystery and awe"

Category 13: Level of Abstractness–Specificity

This category refers to the level at which people identify and describe their strivings. Level can be thought of as existing along a continuum ranging from strivings that are very abstract and reflective at one extreme to strivings that are very concrete and nonreflective at the other extreme. High-level strivings may involve an awareness of internal states (emotions, moods, thoughts), are characterized by self-scrutiny and reflection, and are typically nonbehavioral. Low-level strivings are more likely to be behavioral, less likely to be self reflective or involve self-scrutiny, and are generally more concrete and specific. (Note: Each individual striving can also be rated for level of specification, instead of rating the system as a whole). The scale below is for rating the system as a whole).

Examples of *high-level* strivings:

> "See beyond the myths and illusions that cause many of the symptoms within our society"
> "Find that inner solace and higher mind"
> "Seek new definitions for my life, what is good, desirable, realistic"
> "Use charm and a smiling face to become friends with someone"
> "Do my best in everything I undertake"

Examples of *low-level* strivings:

> "Watch afternoon soap operas"
> "Achieve a 3.0 in my classes"
> "Dress as sharply as possible"

"Avoid fattening foods"
"Keep up household chores"

Use this 5-point scale to rate each person's *list* of strivings (*Note:* You are not
rating each striving separately; you are rating the 15 as a package.)

1	2	3	4	5
more low than high level	equal number high and low	slightly more high than low	many more high than low	almost all high level

References

Affleck, G., Tennen, H., Croog, S., & Levine, S. (1987). Causal attribution, perceived benefits, and morbidity after a heart attack: An 8-year study. *Journal of Consulting and Clinical Psychology, 55,* 29–35.

Affleck, G., Tennen, H., Urrows, S., Higgins, P., Abeles, M., Hall, C., Karoly, P., & Newton, C. (1998). Fibromyalgia and women's pursuit of personal goals: A daily process analysis. *Health Psychology, 17,* 40–47.

Ahuvia, A. C., & Friedman, D. C. (1998). Income, consumption, and subjective well-being: Toward a composite macromarketing model. *Journal of Macromarketing, 18,* 153–168.

Aldwin, C. M. (1994). *Stress, coping, and development: An integrative perspective.* New York: Guilford Press.

Alexander, F. (1950). *Psychosomatic medicine.* New York: Norton.

Allport, F. H. (1937). Teleonomic description in the study of personality. *Character and Personality, 5,* 202–214.

Allport, G. W. (1937). *Personality: A psychological interpretation.* New York: Holt, Rinehart & Winston.

Allport, G. W. (1950). *The individual and his religion.* New York: Macmillan.

Allport, G. W. (1955). *Becoming: Basic considerations for a psychology of personality.* New Haven, CT: Yale University Press.

Anders, T. (1994). *The evolution of evil: An inquiry into the ultimate origins of human suffering.* Chicago: Open Court.

Angyal, A. (1941). *Foundations for a science of personality.* New York: Commonwealth Fund.

Antonovsky, A. (1987). *Unraveling the mystery of health: How people manage stress and stay well.* San Francisco: Jossey-Bass.

Apter, M. J. (1985). Religious states of mind: A reversal theory interpretation. In L. B. Brown (Ed.), *Advances in the psychology of religion* (pp. 62–75). Oxford: Pergamon.

Ashbrook, J. B. (Ed.). (1993). *Brain, culture, and the human spirit: Essays from an emerging evolutionary perspective.* Lanham, MD: University Press of America.

Atchley, R. C. (1995). The continuity of the spiritual self. In S. H. McFadden, M. Kimble, J. W. Ellor, & J. J. Seeber (Eds.), *Aging, spirituality, and religion: A handbook* (pp. 68–73). Minneapolis: Fortress Press.

Atkinson, R. (1995). *The gift of stories*. Westport, CT: Bergin and Garvey.

Augustine. (1960). *The confessions of St. Augustine* (J. K. Ryan,, Trans.). Garden City, NY: Doubleday. (Original work published 397)

Austin, J. T., & Vancouver, J. B. (1996). Goal constructs in psychology: Structure, process, and content. *Psychological Bulletin, 120,* 338–375.

Austin, R. W. J. (1980). *Ibn Al-'Arabi: The bezels of wisdom.* New York: Paulist Press.

Baltes, P. B., & Staudinger, U. M. (1993). The search for a psychology of wisdom. *Current Directions in Psychological Science, 2,* 75–80.

Barbour, I. G. (1960). The methods of science and religion. In H. Shapley (Ed.), *Science ponders religion* (pp. 196–215). New York: Appleton-Century-Crofts.

Bargh, J. A., & Barndollar, K. (1996). Automaticity in action: The unconscious as repository of chronic goals and motives. In P. M. Gollwitzer & J. A. Bargh (Eds.), *The psychology of action: Linking cognition and motivation to behavior* (pp. 457–481). New York: Guilford Press.

Bargh, J. A., & Gollwitzer, P. M. (1994). Environmental control of goal-directed action: Automatic and strategic contingencies between situations and behavior. In W. D. Spaulding (Ed.), *Nebraska Symposium on Motivation* (Vol. 41, pp. 71–124). Lincoln: University of Nebraska Press.

Batson, C. D., & Burris, C. T. (1994). Personal religion: Depressant or stimulant of prejudice and discrimination? In M. P. Zanna & J. M. Olson (Eds.), *The psychology of prejudice: The Ontario symposium, Volume 7* (pp. 149–168). Hillsdale, NJ: Erlbaum.

Batson, C. D., Schoenrade, P., & Ventis, W. L. (1992). *Religion and the individual: A social-psychological perspective.* New York: Oxford University Press.

Baumeister, R. F. (1991). *Meanings of life.* New York: Guilford Press.

Baumeister, R. F., & Exline, J. J. (in press). Virtue, personality, and social relations: Self-control as the moral muscle. *Journal of Personality.*

Baumeister, R. F., & Tice, D. M. (1996). Rethinking and reclaiming the interdisciplary role of personality psychology: The science of human nature should be the center of the social sciences and humanities. *Journal of Research in Personality, 30,* 363–373.

Beit-Hallahmi, B. (1989). *Prolegomena to the psychological study of religion.* Lewisburg, PA: Bucknell University Press.

Berger, P. L. (1967). *The sacred canopy: Elements of a sociological theory of religion.* Garden City, NY: Doubleday.

Bergin, A. E., & Jensen, J. P. (1990). Religiosity of psychotherapists: A national survey. *Psychotherapy, 27,* 3–6.

Bixler, W. G. (1988). Religious legalism. In D. G. Benner (Ed.), *Psychology and religion* (pp. 332–336). Grand Rapids, MI: Baker.

Blaine, B., & Crocker, J. (1995). Religiousness, race, and psychological well-being: Exploring social psychological mediators. *Personality and Social Psychology Bulletin, 21,* 1031–1041.

Blaine, B. E., & Trivedi, P. (1997, August). *Quest religiousness, self-concept integration, and depression.* Paper presented at the annual convention of the American Psychological Association, Chicago.

Blaine, B. E., Trivedi, P., & Eshleman, A. (1998). Religious belief and the self-concept: Evaluating the implications for psychological adjustment. *Personality and Social Psychology Bulletin, 24,* 1040–1052.

Block, J. (1995). A contrarian view of the five-factor approach to personality description. *Psychological Bulletin, 117,* 187–215.

Boisen, A. T. (1936). *The exploration of the inner world.* New York: Harper.

Bowker, J. W. (1976). Information process, systems behavior, and the study of religion. *Zygon, 11, 361–379.*

Brand, J. L. (1997). Challenges for a Christian psychology from cognitive science. *Journal of Psychology and Christianity, 16,* 233–246.

Brandtstadter, J., & Renner, G. (1990). Tenacious goal pursuit and flexible goal adjustment: Explication and age-related analysis of assimilative and accomodative strategies of coping. *Psychology and Aging, 5,* 58–67.

Breed, R. L., & Emmons, R. A. (1996, April). *Personal goals and bereavement: Coping with the loss of a loved one.* Paper presented at the annual convention of the Western Psychological Association, San Jose, CA.

Bregman, L., & Thierman, S. (1995). *First person mortal: Personal narratives of illness, dying, and grief.* New York: Paragon House.

Bridges, C. M., Ware, W. B., Brown, B. B., & Greenwood, G. (1971). Characteristics of the best and worst college teachers. *Science Education, 55,* 545–553.

Brown, D. (1993). The path of meditation: Affective development and psychological well-being. In S. Ablon, D. Brown, E. J. Khantzian, & J. E. Mack (Eds.), *Human feelings: Explorations in affect development and meaning* (pp. 373–402). Hillsdale, NJ: Analytic Press.

Brown, L. B. (Ed.). (1994). *Religion, personality, and mental health.* New York: Springer-Verlag.

Brown, W. S. (1998). Cognitive contributions to soul. In N. Murphy & W. S. Brown, (Eds.), *Portraits of human nature.* (pp. 99–125). Minneapolis: Fortress Press.

Brown, W. S., Murphy, N., & Malony, H. N. (Eds.). (1998). *Whatever happened to the soul?: Scientific and theological portraits of human nature.* Minneapolis: Fortress Press.

Brunstein, J. (1993). Personal goals and subjective well-being: A longitudinal study. *Journal of Personality and Social Psychology, 65,* 1061–1070.

Brunstein, J., Dangelmayer, G., & Schultheiss, O. C. (1996). Personal goals and social support in close relationships: Effects on relationship mood and marital satisfaction. *Journal of Personality and Social Psychology, 71,* 1006–1019.

Brunstein, J. C., Schultheiss, O. C., & Graessman, R. (1998). Personal goals and emotional well-being: The moderating role of motive dispositions. *Journal of Personality and Social Psychology, 75,* 494–508.

Burhoe, R. W. (1981). *Toward a scientific theology.* Belfast, Northern Ireland: Christian Journals Limited.

Buss, D. M. (1995). Evolutionary psychology: A new paradigm for psychological science. *Psychological Inquiry, 6,* 1–30.

Call, V. R., & Heaton, T. B. (1997). Religious influence on marital stability. *Journal for the Scientific Study of Religion, 36,* 382–392.

Calvin, J. (1984). *The Christian life* (J. H. Leith, Ed.). San Francisco: Harper & Row. (Original work published 1559)

Cantor, N. (1990). From thought to behavior: "Having" and "doing" in the study of personality and cognition. *American Psychologist, 45,* 735–750.

Cantor, N., & Kihlstrom, J. (1987). *Personality and social intelligence.* Englewood Cliffs, NJ: Prentice-Hall.

Cantor, N., & Langston, C. A. (1989). Ups and downs of life tasks in a life transition. In L. A. Pervin (Ed.), *Goal concepts in personality and social psychology* (pp. 127–167). Hillsdale, NJ: Erlbaum.

Cantor, N., & Zirkel, S. (1990). Personality, cognition, and purposive behavior. In L. A. Pervin (Ed.), *Handbook of personality: Theory and research* (pp. 135–164). New York: Guilford Press.

Caprara, G. V. (1996). Reflections on the scientific status and perspectives of personality psychology. In J. Georgas, M. Manthouli, E. Besevegis, & A. Kokkevi (Eds.), *Contemporary psychology in Europe* (pp. 103–117). Seattle: Hogrefe & Huber.

Carver, C. S., & Scheier, M. F. (1998). *On the self-regulation of behavior.* New York: Cambridge University Press.

Carver, C. S., & White, T. L. (1994). Behavioral inhibition, behavioral activation, and affective responses to impending reward and punishment: The BIS/BAS scales. *Journal of Personality and Social Psychology, 67,* 319–333.

Chamberlain, K., & Zika, S. (1992). Religiosity, meaning in life, and psychological well-being. In J. F. Schumaker (Ed.), *Religion and mental health* (pp. 138–148). New York: Oxford University Press.

Chiu, C., Hong, Y., & Dweck, C. S. (1994). Toward an integrative model of personality and intelligence: A general framework and some preliminary steps. In R. J. Sternberg & P. Ruzgis (Eds.), *Personality and intelligence* (pp. 104–134). New York: Cambridge University Press.

Chulef, A. S., Read, S. J., & Walsh, D. A. (1996). *A hierarchical taxonomy of human goals.* Unpublished manuscript, University of Southern California, Los Angeles.

Clark, A. T. (1992). Humility. In D. H. Ludlow (Ed.), *Encyclopedia of Mormonism* (pp. 663–664). New York: Macmillan.

Clark, W. H. (1958). *The psychology of religion.* New York: Macmillan.

Cloninger, S. C. (1996). *Personality: Description, dynamics, and development.* New York: Freeman.

Coats, E. J., Janoff-Bulman, R., & Alpert, N. (1996). Approach versus avoidance goals: Differences in self-evaluation and well-being. *Personality and Social Psychology Bulletin, 22,* 1057–1067.

Cochran, W., & Tesser, A. (1996). Some effects of goal proximity and goal framing on performance. In L. L. Martin & A. Tesser (Eds.), *Striving and feeling: Interactions among goals, affect, and self-regulation* (pp. 99–120). Mahwah, NJ: Erlbaum.

Colby, A., & Damon, W. (1992). *Some do care: Contemporary lives of moral commitment.* New York: Free Press.

Colby, P. M. (1996). *Individual differences in identity development status: Social and cognitive correlates of goal integration in early adulthood.* Unpublished doctoral dissertation, University of California, Davis.

Compton, W. C., Smith, M. L., Cornish, K. A., & Qualls, D. L. (1996). Factor structure of mental health measures. *Journal of Personality and Social Psychology, 71,* 406–413.

Cox, W. M., & Klinger, E. (1988). A motivational model of alcohol use. *Journal of Abnormal Psychology, 97,* 168–180.

Crabtree, H. (1991). *The Christian life: Traditional metaphors and contemporary theologies.* Minneapolis: Fortress Press.

Craik, K. H., & Hogan, R. (Eds.). (1993). *Fifty years of personality psychology.* New York: Plenum.

Csikszentmihalyi, M. (1990). *Flow: The psychology of optimal experience.* New York: HarperCollins.

Csikszentmihalyi, M. (1993). *The evolving self.* New York: HarperCollins.

Danielou, J., & Musurillo, H. (Eds.). (1961). *From glory to glory: Texts from Gregory of Nyssa's mystical writings.* New York: Scribner's.

d'Aquili, E. G., & Newberg, A. B. (1998). The neuropsychological basis of religion, or why God won't go away. *Zygon, 33,* 187–202.

Davidson, J. C., & Caddell, D. P. (1994). Religion and the meaning of work. *Journal for the Scientific Study of Religion, 33,* 135–147.

Deci, E. L., & Ryan, R. M. (1985). *Intrinsic motivation and self-determination in human behavior.* New York: Plenum.

Deci, E. L., & Ryan, R. M. (1991). A motivational approach to self: Integration in personality. In R. A. Dienstbier (Ed.), *Nebraska Symposium on Motivation* (Vol. 38, pp. 237–288). Lincoln: University of Nebraska Press.

DeNeve, K. M., & Cooper, H. (1998). The happy personality: A meta-analysis of 137 personality traits and subjective well-being. *Psychological Bulletin, 124,* 197–229.

Descutner, C. J., & Thelen, M. H. (1991). Development and validation of a fear of intimacy scale. *Psychological Assessment: A Journal of Consulting and Clinical Psychology, 3,* 218–225.

Diener, E. (1984). Subjective well-being. *Psychological Bulletin, 95,* 542–575.

Diener, E. (1995). Assessing subjective well-being: Opportunities and progress. *Social Indicators Research, 31,* 103–157.

Diener, E. (1996). Traits can be powerful, but are not enough: Lessons from subjective well-being. *Journal of Research in Personality, 30,* 389–399.

Diener, E., & Diener, C. (1996). Most people are happy. *Psychological Science, 7,* 181–186.

Diener, E., & Emmons, R. A. (1984). The independence of positive and negative affect. *Journal of Personality and Social Psychology, 47,* 1105–1117.

Diener, E., Emmons, R., Larsen, R., & Griffin, S. (1985). The Satisfaction with Life Scale. *Journal of Personality Assessment, 49,* 71–75.

Diener, E., & Fujita, F. (1995). Resources, personal strivings, and subjective well-being: A nomothetic and idiographic approach. *Journal of Personality and Social Psychology, 68,* 926–935.

Digman, J. M. (1990). Personality structure: Emergence of the five-factor model. *Annual Review of Psychology, 41,* 417–440.

Dittes, J. (1968). Psychology of religion. In G. Lindzey & E. Aronson (Eds.), *The handbook of social psychology* (2nd ed., Vol. 5, pp. 602–659). Reading, MA: Addison-Wesley.

Dixon, J. P., & Dixon, J. K. (1991). Contradictory tendencies in the perception of life conflicts in persons with cardiovascular disease and persons with cancer. *Personality and Individual Differences, 12,* 791–799.

Dixon, R. A., & Baltes, P. B. (1986). Toward life span research on the functions and pragmatics of intelligence. In R. J. Sternberg & R. K. Wagner (Eds.), *Practical intelligence: Nature and origins of competence in the everyday world* (pp. 203–235). New York: Cambridge University Press.

Dollahite, D. C. (1998). Fathering, faith, and spirituality. *Journal of Men's Studies, 7,* 3–15.

Dollahite, D. C., Slife, B., Hawkins, A. J. (1997). Family generativity and generative counseling: Helping families keep faith with the next generation. In D. P. McAdams & E. St. Aubin (Eds.), *Generativity and adult development: Psychological perspectives on caring for and contributing to the next generation* (pp. 449–481). Washington, DC: American Psychological Association.

Donahue, E. M., Robins, R. W., Roberts, B. W., & John, O. P. (1993). The divided self: Concurrent and longitudinal effects of psychological adjustment and social roles on self-concept differentiation. *Journal of Personality and Social Psychology, 64,* 834–846.

Dramatic rise seen in those who say religion increasing influence. *Emerging Trends, 20*(4, 5), 1.

Dweck, C. S. (1990). Self-theories and goals: Their role in motivation, personality, and development. In R. A. Dienstbier (Ed.), *Nebraska Symposium on Motivation* (Vol. 38, pp. 199–235). Lincoln: University of Nebraska Press.

Edmonds, S., & Hooker, K. (1992). Perceived changes in life meaning following bereavement. *Omega, 25,* 307-318.

Edwards, J. (1959). *A treatise concerning religious affections* (J. E. Smith, Ed.). New Haven, CT: Yale University Press. (Original work published 1746)

Ehrenberg, M. F., Hunter, M. A., & Elterman, M. F. (1996). Shared parenting agreements after marital separation: The roles of empathy and narcissism. *Journal of Consulting and Clinical Psychology, 64,* 808–818.

Elkins, D. N. (1988). Towards a humanistic–phenomenological spirituality: Definition, description, and measurement. *Journal of Humanistic Psychology, 28,* 5–18.

Elliot, A. J., & Sheldon, K. M. (1997). Avoidance achievement motivation: A personal goals analysis. *Journal of Personality and Social Psychology, 73,* 171–185.

Elliot, A. J., & Sheldon, K. M. (1998). Avoidance, personal goals and the personality–illness relationship. *Journal of Personality and Social Psychology, 75,* 1282–1299.

Elliot, A. J., Sheldon, K. M., & Church, M. (1997). Avoidance personal goals and subjective well-being. *Personality and Social Psychology Bulletin, 23,* 915–927.

Ellis, A. (1980). Psychotherapy and atheistic values: A response to A. E. Bergin's

"Psychotherapy and Religious Values." *Journal of Consulting and Clinical Psychology, 48,* 635–639.

Ellison, C. W. (1983). Spiritual well-being: Conceptualization and measurement. *Journal of Psychology and Theology, 11,* 330–340.

Ellison, C. W., & Smith, J. (1991). Toward an integrative measure of health and well-being. *Journal of Psychology and Theology, 19,* 35–48.

Emmons, R. A. (1986). Personal strivings: An approach to personality and subjective well-being. *Journal of Personality and Social Psychology, 51,* 1058–1068.

Emmons, R. A. (1989). The personal striving approach to personality. In L. A. Pervin (Ed.), *Goal concepts in personality and social psychology* (pp. 87–126). Hillsdale, NJ: Erlbaum.

Emmons, R. A. (1991). Personal strivings, daily life events, and psychological and physical well-being. *Journal of Personality, 59,* 453–472.

Emmons, R. A. (1992). Abstract versus concrete goals: Personal striving level, physical illness, and psychological well-being. *Journal of Personality and Social Psychology, 62,* 292–300.

Emmons, R. A. (1993). Current status of the motive concept. In K. H. Craik, R. Hogan, & R. N. Wolfe (Eds.), *Fifty years of personality psychology* (pp. 187–196). New York: Plenum.

Emmons, R. A. (1996). Striving and feeling: Personal goals and subjective well-being. In P. M. Gollwitzer & J. A. Bargh (Eds.), *The psychology of action: Linking cognition and motivation to behavior* (pp. 313–337). New York: Guilford Press.

Emmons, R. A. (1997). Motives and life goals. In R. Hogan, J. Johnson, & S. Briggs (Eds.), *Handbook of personality psychology* (pp. 485–512). San Diego, CA: Academic Press.

Emmons, R. A., Cheung, C., & Tehrani, K. (1998). Assessing spirituality through personal goals: Implications for research on religion and subjective well-being. *Social Indicators Research, 45,* 391–422.

Emmons, R. A., & Colby, P. M. (1995). Emotional conflict and well-being: Relation to perceived availability, daily utilization, and observer reports of social support. *Journal of Personality and Social Psychology, 68,* 947–959.

Emmons, R. A., Colby, P. M., & Kaiser, H. A. (1998). When losses lead to gains: Personal goals and the recovery of meaning. In P. T. P. Wong & P. S. Fry (Eds.), *The human quest for meaning* (pp. 163–178). Mahwah, NJ: Erlbaum.

Emmons, R. A., & Crumpler, C. A. (in press). Gratitude as a human strength: Appraising the evidence. *Journal of Social and Clinical Psychology.*

Emmons, R. A., & Kaiser, H. (1996). Goal orientation and emotional well-being: Linking goals and affect through the self. In A. Tesser & L. Martin (Eds.), *Striving and feeling: Interactions among goals, affect, and self-regulation* (pp. 79–98). New York: Plenum.

Emmons, R. A., & King, L. A. (1988). Conflict among personal strivings: Immediate and long-term implications for psychological and physical well-being. *Journal of Personality and Social Psychology, 54,* 1040–1048.

Emmons, R. A., & King, L. A. (1989). Personal striving differentiation and affective reactivity. *Journal of Personality and Social Psychology, 56,* 478–484.

Emmons, R. A., King, L. A., & Sheldon, K. (1993). Goal conflict and the self-regulation of action. In D. M. Wegner & J. W. Pennebaker (Eds), *Handbook of mental control* (pp. 528–551). Englewood Cliffs, NJ: Prentice-Hall.

Emmons, R. A., & McAdams, D. P. (1991). Personal strivings and motive dispositions: Exploring the links. *Personality and Social Psychology Bulletin, 17,* 648–654.

Epstein, S. (1982). Conflict and stress. In L. Goldberger & S. Breznitz (Eds.), *Handbook of stress* (pp. 49–68). New York: Free Press.

Epstein, S. (1991). The self-concept, the traumatic neurosis, and the structure of personality. In D. J. Ozer, J. M. Healy, Jr., & A. J. Stewart (Eds.), *Perspectives in personality* (Vol. 3A, pp. 63–98). London: Kingsley.

Epstein, S. (1993). *You're smarter than you think: How to develop your practical intelligence for success in living.* New York: Simon & Schuster.

Epstein, S. (1994). Integration of the cognitive and psychodynamic unconscious. *American Psychologist, 49,* 709–724.

Erickson, M. J. (1985). *Christian theology.* Grand Rapids, MI: Baker Book House.

Erikson, E. H. (1950). *Childhood and society.* New York: Norton.

Ewart, C. K. (1991). Social action theory for a public health psychology. *American Psychologist, 46,* 931–946.

Ewart, C. K. (1994). Nonshared environments and heart disease risk: Concepts and data for a model of coronary-prone behavior. In E. Heatherington, D. Reiss, & R. Plomin (Eds.), *Separate social worlds of siblings: The impact of nonshared environment on development* (pp. 175–204). Hillsdale, NJ: Erlbaum.

Fichter, J. H. (1981). *Religion and pain: Spiritual dimensions of health care.* New York: Crossroad.

Finger, T. N. (1997). *Self, earth, and society: Alienation and trinitarian transformation.* Downers Grove, IL: InterVarsity Press.

Foerst, A. (1996). Artificial intelligence: Walking the boundary. *Zygon, 31,* 681–693.

Folkman, S., & Stein, N. L. (1997). Adaptive goal processes in stressful events. In N. Stein, P. A. Ornstein, B. Tversky, & C. Brainerd (Eds.), *Memory for everyday and emotional events* (pp. 113–137). Hillsdale, NJ: Erlbaum.

Ford, D., & Nichols, (1987). A taxonomy of human goals and some possible applications. In M. E. Ford & D. H. Ford (Eds.), *Humans as self-constructing living systems: Putting the framework to work* (pp. 289–311). Hillsdale, NJ: Erlbaum.

Ford, M. E. (1992). *Motivating humans: Goals, emotions, and personal agency beliefs.* Newbury Park, CA: Sage.

Ford, M. E. (1994). A living systems approach to the integration of personality and intelligence. In R. J. Sternberg & P. Ruzgis (Eds.), *Personality and intelligence* (pp. 188–217). New York: Cambridge University Press.

Fosdick, H. E. (1943). *On being a real person.* New York: Harper & Row.

Fowler, J. W. (1981). *Stages of faith: The psychology of human development and the quest for meaning.* New York: HarperCollins.

Franz, C., & Stewart, A. J. (Eds.). (1994). *Women creating lives: Identities, resilience, and resistance.* Boulder, CO: Westview.

Frese, M., & Sabini, J. (Eds.). (1985). *Goal-directed behavior: The concept of action in psychology*. Hillsdale, NJ: Erlbaum.

Freund, A. M., & Baltes, P. B. (1998). Selection, optimization, and compensation as strategies of life management: Correlations with subjective indicators of successful aging. *Psychology and Aging, 13,* 531–543.

Friedman, H. S., & Booth-Kewley, S. (1987). The "disease-prone personality": A meta-analytic view of the construct. *American Psychologist, 42,* 539–555.

Gallup, G. H., Jr., & Castelli, J. (1989). *The people's religion: American faith in the 90's.* New York: Macmillan.

Gardner, H. (1993). *Frames of mind* (10th anniversary ed.). New York: Basic Books.

Gardner, H. (1995, November). Reflections on multiple intelligences: Myths and messages. *Phi Delta Kappan,* 204–207.

Gardner, H. (1996, November). Probing more deeply into the theory of multiple intelligences. *NASSP Bulletin,* 1–7.

Gardner, H. (in press). Are there additional intelligences? The case for naturalist, spiritual, and existential intelligences. In J. Kane (Ed.), *Education, information, and transformation.* Englewood Cliffs, NJ: Prentice-Hall.

Gartner, J. (1996). Religious commitments, mental health, and prosocial behavior: A review of the empirical literature. In E. F. Shafranske (Ed.), *Religion and the clinical practice of psychology* (pp. 187–214). Washington, DC: American Psychological Association.

Geertz, C. (1966). Religion as a cultural system. In M. Benton (Ed.), *Anthropological approaches to the study of religion* (pp. 1–46). London: Tavistock.

Gilbert, D. T., Fiske, S. T., & Lindzey, G. (Eds.). (1997). *Handbook of social psychology* (4th ed.). Boston: McGraw-Hill.

Glock, C. Y. (1962). On the study of religious commitment. *Religious Education, 57,* 98–109.

Glock, C. Y., & Stark, R. (1965). *Religion and society in tension.* Chicago: Rand-McNally.

Gollwitzer, P. M. (1993). Goal achievement: The role of intentions. In W. Stroebe & M. Hewstone (Eds.), *European review of social psychology* (Vol. 4, pp. 141–185). Chichester, England: Wiley.

Gollwitzer, P. M., & Bargh, J. A. (Eds.). (1996). *The psychology of action: Linking cognition and motivation to behavior.* New York: Guilford Press.

Gomersall, T. E. (1993). *Personal strivings and repression: Identifying the repressive coping style within the personal strivings framework.* Unpublished master's thesis, Humboldt State University, Arcata, CA.

Gorsuch, R. L. (1984). Measurement: The boon and bane of investigating religion. *American Psychologist, 39,* 228–236.

Gorsuch, R. L., & McPherson, S. E. (1989). Intrinsic/extrinsic measurement: I/E revised and single-item scales. *Journal for the Scientific Study of Religion, 28,* 348–354.

Gray, J. A. (1987). *The psychology of fear and stress.* New York: Cambridge University Press.

Greenberg, L. S., & Safran, J. D. (1987). *Emotion in psychotherapy.* New York: Guilford Press.

Hall, T. W., & Edwards, K. J. (1996). The initial development and factor analysis of the spiritual assessment inventory. *Journal of Psychology and Theology, 24*, 233–246.

Haslam, N., & Baron, J. (1994). Intelligence, prudence, and personality. In R. J. Sternberg & P. Ruzgis (Eds.), *Personality and intelligence* (pp. 32–58). New York: Cambridge University Press.

Hawkins, A. J., & Dollahite, D. C. (Eds.). (1997). *Generative fathering: Beyond deficit perspectives* (pp. 17–35). Thousand Oaks, CA: Sage.

Heatherton, T., & Weinberger, J. (Eds.). (1994). *Does personality change?* Washington, DC: American Psychological Association.

Hefner, P. (1993). *The human factor.* Minneapolis: Fortress Press.

Heitler, S. M. (1990). *From conflict to resolution.* New York: Norton.

Herman, J. L. (1992). *Trauma and recovery.* New York: Basic Books.

Heschel, A. (1955). *God in search of man: A philosophy of Judaism.* New York: Farrar, Strauss, & Cudahy.

Higgins, E. T. (1987). Self-discrepancy: A theory relating self and affect. *Psychological Review, 94*, 319–340.

Hill, P. C. (in press). Giving religion away: What the study of religion offers psychology. *International Journal for the Psychology of Religion.*

Hogan, R. (1976). *Personality theory: The personological tradition.* Englewood Cliffs, NJ: Prentice-Hall.

Hogan, R., Johnson, J., & Briggs, S. (Eds.). (1997). *Handbook of personality psychology.* San Diego, CA: Academic Press.

Hood, R. W., Jr., Spilka, B., Hunsberger, B., & Gorsuch, R. (1996). *The psychology of religion: An empirical approach* (2nd ed.). New York: Guilford Press.

Hyland, M. E. (1988). Motivational control theory: An integrative framework. *Journal of Personality and Social Psychology, 55*, 642–651.

Inglehart, R. (1990). *Culture shift in advanced industrial society.* Princeton, NJ: Princeton University Press.

Ingram, J. A. (1996). Psychological aspects of the filling of the Holy Spirit: A preliminary model of post-redemptive personality functioning. *Journal of Psychology and Theology, 24*, 104–113.

James, W. (1902). *The varieties of religious experience.* New York: Longman.

Janis, I. L., Mahl, G. F., Kagan, J., & Holt, R. R. (1969). *Personality: Development, dynamics, and change.* New York: Harcourt, Brace, and World.

Janis, I. L., & Mann, L. (1977). *Decision making: A psychological analysis of conflict, choice, and commitment.* New York: Free Press.

Jeeves, M. A. (1997). *Human nature at the millennium.* Grand Rapids, MI: Baker Books.

Jockin, V., McGue, M., & Lykken, D. T. (1996). Personality and divorce: A genetic analysis. *Journal of Personality and Social Psychology, 71*, 288–299.

Jurors prefer lawyers who are well-prepared—and not arrogant. (1993, February 22). *National Law Journal, 15*, 10.

Karoly, P. (1991). Goal systems and health outcomes across the life span: A proposal. In H. E. Schroeder (Ed.), *New directions in health psychology assessment* (pp. 65–91). New York: Hemisphere.

Karoly, P. (1993). Goal systems: An organizational framework for clinical assessment and treatment planning. *Psychological Assessment, 3,* 273-280.

Karoly, P., & Bay, R. C. (1990). Diabetes self-care goals and their relation to children's metabolic control. *Journal of Pediatric Psychology, 15,* 83–95.

Karoly, P. & McKeeman, D. (1991). Interpersonal and intrapsychic goal-related conflict reported by cigarette smokers, unaided quitters, and relapsers. *Addictive Behaviors, 16,* 543–548.

Karoly, P., & Ruehlman, L. S. (1996). Motivational implications of pain: Chronicity, psychological distress, and work goal construal in a national sample of adults. *Health Psychology, 15,* 383–390.

Kasser, T., & Ryan, R. M. (1993). A dark side of the American dream: Correlates of financial success as a central life aspiration. *Journal of Personality and Social Psychology, 65,* 410–422.

Kasser, T., & Ryan, R. M. (1996). Further examining the American dream: The differential effects of intrinsic and extrinsic goal structures. *Personality and Social Psychology Bulletin, 22,* 280–287.

Katz, I. M., & Campbell, J. D. (1994). Ambivalence over emotional expression and well-being: Nomothetic and idiographic tests of the stress-buffering hypothesis. *Journal of Personality and Social Psychology, 67,* 513–524.

Keany, K. C., & Glueckauf, R. L. (1993). Disability and value change: An overview and reanalysis of acceptance of loss theory. *Rehabilitation Psychology, 38,* 199–210.

Kelly, E. W., Jr. (1995). *Spirituality and religion in counseling and psychotherapy.* Alexandria, VA: American Counseling Association.

Kendler, K. S., Gardner, C. O., & Prescott, C. A. (1997). Religion, psychopathology, and substance use and abuse: A multimeasure, genetic-epidemiologic study. *American Journal of Psychiatry, 154,* 322–329.

King, L. A. (1993). Emotional expression, conflict over expression, and marital satisfaction. *Journal of Social and Personal Relationships, 10,* 601–607.

King, L. A. (1995). Wishes, motives, goals, and personal memories: Relations of measures of human motivation. *Journal of Personality, 63,* 985–1007.

King, L. A. (1998). Ambivalence over emotional expression and reading emotions in situations and faces. *Journal of Personality and Social Psychology, 74,* 753–762.

King, L. A., & Emmons, R. A. (1990). Conflict over emotional expression: Psychological and physical correlates. *Journal of Personality and Social Psychology, 58,* 864–877.

King, L. A., & Emmons, R. A. (1991). Psychological, physical, and interpersonal correlates of emotional expressiveness, conflict, and control. *European Journal of Personality, 5,* 131–150.

King, L. A., Emmons, R. A., & Woodley, S. (1992). The structure of inhibition. *Journal of Research in Personality, 26,* 85–102.

King, L. A., & Napa, C. K. (1998). What makes a life good? *Journal of Personality and Social Psychology, 75,* 156–165.

King, L. A., Richards, J. H., & Stemmerich, E. (1998). Daily goals, life goals, and worst fears: Means, ends, and subjective well-being. *Journal of Personality, 66,* 713–744.

King, V., & Elder, G. H., Jr. (1998, August). *Are religious grandparents more involved grandparents?* Paper presented at the annual convention of the American Sociological Association, San Francisco, CA.

Kirkpatrick, L. A. (in press). Toward an evolutionary psychology of religion and personality. *Journal of Personality.*

Kirkpatrick, L., & Hood, R. W., Jr. (1990). Intrinsic–extrinsic religious orientation: The "boon" or "bane" of contemporary psychology of religion? *Journal for the Scientific Study of Religion, 29,* 442–462.

Klinger, E. (1977). *Meaning and void: Inner experience and the incentives in people's lives.* Minneapolis, MN: University of Minnesota Press.

Klinger, E. (1987). The interview questionnaire technique: Reliability and validity of a mixed idiographic–nomothetic measure of motivation. In J. N. Butcher & C. D. Spielberger (Eds.), *Advances in personality assessment* (Vol. 6, pp. 31–48). Hillsdale, NJ: Erlbaum.

Klinger, E. (1998). The search for meaning in evolutionary perspective and its clinical implications. In P. T. P. Wong & P. S. Fry (Eds.), *The human quest for meaning* (pp. 27–50). Mahwah, NJ: Erlbaum.

Kluckhohn, C., & Murray, H. A. (1953). Outline of a conception of personality. In H. A. Murray and C. Kluckhohn, *Personality in nature, society, and culture* (2nd ed., pp. 3–32). New York: Knopf.

Koenig, H. G. (1997). *Is religion good for your health? The effects of religion on physical and mental health.* Binghamton, NY: Haworth Press.

Koenig, H. G. (Ed.). (1998). *Handbook of religion and mental health.* San Diego, CA: Academic Press.

Kojetin, B. A., McIntosh, D. N., Bridges, R. A., & Spilka, B. (1987). Quest: Constructive search or religious conflict? *Journal for the Scientific Study of Religion, 26,* 111–115.

Kovac, D. (1996). Quality of the environment and quality of life. In J. Georgas (Ed.), *Contemporary psychology in Europe: Theory, research, and applications* (pp. 184–193). Seattle, WA: Hogrefe & Huber.

Kramer, D. A. (1990). Conceptualizing wisdom: The primacy of affect-cognition relations. In R. J. Sternberg (Ed.), *Wisdom: Its nature, origins, and development* (pp. 121–141). New York: Cambridge University Press.

Kreitler, S., & Chemerinski, A. (1988). The cognitive orientation of obesity. *International Journal of Obesity, 12,* 403–415.

Kreitler, S., & Kreitler, H. (1991). Cognitive orientation and physical disease or health. *European Journal of Personality, 5,* 109–129.

Kruglanski, A. W. (1996). Goals as knowledge structures. In P. M. Gollwitzer & J. A. Bargh (Eds.), *The psychology of action: Linking cognition and motivation to behavior* (pp. 599–618). New York: Guilford Press.

Lapierre, S., Bouffard, L., & Bastin, E. (1997). Personal goals and subjective well-being in later life. *International Journal of Aging and Human Development, 45,* 287–302.

Lauterbach, W. (1975). Covariation of conflict and mood in depression. *British Journal of Clinical and Social Psychology, 14,* 49–53.

Lauterbach, W. (1990). Intrapersonal conflict, life stress, and emotion. In C. D.

Spielberger, I. G. Sarason, J. Strelau, & J. M. T. Brebner (Eds.), *Stress and anxiety* (Vol. 3, pp. 85–92). New York: Hemisphere.

Lavallee, L. F., & Campbell, J. D. (1995). Impact of personal goals on self-regulation processes elicited by daily negative events. *Journal of Personality and Social Psychology, 69,* 341–352.

Lawler, J. E., Barker, G. F., Hubbard, J. W., & Allen, M. T. (1980). The effects of conflict on tonic levels of blood pressure in the genetically borderline hypertensive rat. *Psychophysiology, 17,* 363–370.

Lawton, M. P. (1996). Quality of life and affect in later life. In C. Magai & S. H. McFadden (Eds.), *Handbook of emotion, adult development and aging* (pp. 327–348). San Diego, CA: Academic Press.

Lazarus, R. S. (1991). *Emotion and adaptation.* New York: Oxford University Press.

Lazarus, R. S. (1993). Coping theory and research: Past, present, and future. *Psychosomatic Medicine, 55,* 234–247.

Lazarus, R. S., & Folkman, S. (1984). *Stress, appraisal, and coping.* New York: Springer.

Lecci, L., Karoly, P., Briggs, C., & Kuhn, K. (1994). Specificity and generality of motivational components in depression: A personal projects analysis. *Journal of Abnormal Psychology, 103,* 404–408.

Lecci, L., Karoly, P., Ruehlman, L. S., & Lanyon, R. I. (1996). Goal-relevant dimensions of hypochondriacal tendencies and their relation to symptom manifestation and psychologic distress. *Journal of Abnormal Psychology, 105,* 42–52.

Lecci, L., Okun, O., & Karoly, P. (1994). Life regrets and current goals as predictors of psychological adjustment. *Journal of Personality and Social Psychology, 66,* 731–741.

Lester, D. (1995). *Theories of personality: A systems approach.* Washington, DC: Taylor & Francis.

Levenson, M. R., & Crumpler, C. (1996). Three models of adult development. *Human Development, 39,* 135–149.

Levin, J. S., & Tobin, S. S. (1995). Religion and psychological well-being. In M. A. Kimble, S. H. McFadden, J. W. Ellor, & J. J. Seeber (Eds.), *Aging, spirituality, and religion: A handbook* (pp. 30–46). Minneapolis, MN: Fortress Press.

Lewis, C. S. (1960). *Mere Christianity.* New York: Macmillan.

Lewis, C. S. (1970). *The grand miracle.* New York: Ballantine.

Lickona, T. (1991). *Educating for character: How are schools can teach respect and responsibility.* New York: Bantam Books.

Lifton, R. J. (1979). *The broken connection: On death and the continuity of life.* New York: Simon & Schuster.

Lifton, R. J. (1993). *The protean self: Human resilience in an age of fragmentation.* New York: Basic Books.

Little, B. R. (1989). Personal projects analysis: Trivial pursuits, magnificent obsessions, and the search for coherence. In D. M. Buss & N. Cantor (Eds.), *Personality psychology: Recent trends and emerging directions* (pp. 15–31). New York: Springer-Verlag.

Little, B. R. (1993). Personal projects and the distributed self: Aspects of a conative psychology. In J. Suls (Ed.), *Psychological perspectives on the self* (Vol. 4, pp. 157–181). Hillsdale, NJ: Erlbaum.

Little, B. R. (1996). Free traits, personal projects, and idio-tapes: Three tiers for personality psychology. *Psychological Inquiry, 7,* 340–344.

Little, D. (1989). Human suffering in comparative perspective. In R. L. Taylor & J. Watson (Eds.), *They shall not hurt: Human suffering and human caring* (pp. 53–72). Boulder, CO: Colorado Associated University Press.

The Living Bible. (1988). Wheaton, IL: Tyndale House.

Locke, E. A., & Kristof, A. L. (1996). Volitional choices in the goal achievement process. In P. M. Gollwitzer & J. A. Bargh (Eds.), *The psychology of action: Linking cognition and motivation to behavior* (pp. 365–384). New York: Guilford Press.

Loehlin, J. (1992). *Genes and environment in personality development.* Beverly Hills, CA: Sage.

Loevinger, J. (1976). *Ego development.* San Francisco: Jossey-Bass.

Lucas, R. E., Diener, E., & Suh, E. (1996). Discriminant validity of well-being measures. *Journal of Personality and Social Psychology, 71,* 616–628.

Luther, M. (1957). *The bondage of the will* (J. I. Parker & O. R. Johnston, Trans.). Westwood, NJ: Revell. (Original work published 1525)

Lykken, D. T., & Tellegen, A. (1996). Happiness is a stochastic phenomenon. *Psychological Science, 7,* 186–189.

MacDonald, K. (1995). Evolution, the five-factor model, and personality. *Journal of Personality, 63,* 525–568.

Mahoney, A., Pargament, K. I., Jewell, T., Swank, A. B., Scott, E., Emery, E., & Rye, M. (in press). Marriage and the spiritual realm: The roles of proximal and distal religious constructs in marital functioning. *Journal of Family Psychology.*

Malony, N. (1988). The clinical assessment of optimal religious functioning. *Review of Religious Research, 30,* 3–17.

Marsden, G. M. (1997). *The outrageous idea of Christian scholarship.* New York: Oxford University Press.

Martin, J. E., & Carlson, C. R. (1988). Spiritual dimensions of health psychology. In W. R. Miller & J. E. Martin (Eds.), *Behavior therapy and religion: Integrating spiritual and behavioral approaches to change* (pp. 57–110). Newbury Park, CA: Sage.

Martin, L. L., & Tesser, A. (Eds.). (1996). *Striving and feeling: Interactions among goals, affect, and self-regulation.* Hillsdale, NJ: Erlbaum.

Maslow, A. (1955). Deficiency motivation and growth motivation. In M. R. Jones (Ed.), *Nebraska Symposium on Motivation* (Vol. 3, pp. 1–30). Lincoln: University of Nebraska Press.

Maton, K. I. (1989). The stress-buffering role of spiritual support: Cross-sectional and prospective investigations. *Journal for the Scientific Study of Religion, 28,* 310–323.

Mayer, J. D., & Salovey, P. (1997). What is emotional intelligence? In P. Salovey & D. J. Sluyter (Eds.), *Emotional development and emotional intelligence* (pp. 3–31). New York: Basic Books.

McAdams, D. P. (1989). *Intimacy: The need to be close.* New York: Doubleday.

McAdams, D. P. (1992). The five-factor model in personality: A critical appraisal. *Journal of Personality, 60,* 329–361.

McAdams, D. P. (1993). *The stories we live by: Personal myths and the making of the self.* New York: Morrow.

McAdams, D. P. (1995). What do we know when we know a person? *Journal of Personality, 63,* 365–396.

McAdams, D. P. (1996). Personality, modernity, and the storied self: A contemporary framework for studying persons. *Psychological Inquiry, 7,* 295–321.

McAdams, D. P. (1997). A conceptual history of personal psychology. In R. Hogan, J. Johnson, & S. Briggs (Eds.), *Handbook of personality psychology* (pp. 3–39). San Diego, CA: Academic Press.

McAdams, D. P., & de St. Aubin, E. (1992). A theory of generativity and its assessment through self-report, behavioral acts, and narrative themes in autobiography. *Journal of Personality and Social Psychology, 62,* 1003-1015.

McAdams, D. P., & de St. Aubin, E. (Eds.). (1998). *Generativity and adult development: Psychosocial perspectives on caring for and contributing to the next generation.* Washington, DC: American Psychological Association.

McClelland, D. C. (1985). *Human motivation.* Glenview, IL: Scott, Foresman.

McClelland, D. C. (1989). Motivational factors in health and disease. *American Psychologist, 44,* 675-683.

McClelland, D. C., Koestner, R., & Weinberger, J. (1989). How do self-attributed and implicit motives differ? *Psychological Review, 96,* 690–702.

McClennon, J. (1997). Shamanic healing, human evolution, and the origin of religion. *Journal for the Scientific Study of Religion, 36,* 345–354.

McCrae, R. R., & Costa, P. T., Jr. (1990). *Personality in adulthood.* New York: Guilford Press.

McCrae, R. R., & Costa, P. T., Jr. (1996). Toward a new generation of personality theories: Theoretical contexts for the five-factor model. In J. S. Wiggins (Ed.), *The five-factor model of personality: Theoretical perspectives* (pp. 51 87). New York: Guilford Press.

McCullough, M. E. (1995). Prayer and health: Conceptual issues, research review, and research agenda. *Journal of Psychology and Theology, 23,* 15–29.

McGregor, I., & Little, B. R. (1998). Personal projects, happiness, and meaning: On doing well and being yourself. *Journal of Personality and Social Psychology, 74,* 494–512.

McIntosh, D., Silver, R., & Wortman, C. (1993). Religion's role in adjustment to a negative life event: Coping with the loss of a child. *Journal of Personality and Social Psychology, 65,* 812–821.

McReynolds, P. (1990). The nature and logic of intrapsychic conflicts. In C. D. Spielberger, I. G. Sarason, J. Strelau, & J. M. T. Brebner (Eds.), *Stress and anxiety* (Vol. 3, pp. 73–83). New York: Hemisphere.

Meehl, P. E. (1964). *Manual for use with checklist of schizotypic signs.* Minneapolis: University of Minnesota Medical School, Psychiatric Research Unit.

Megargee, E. (1997). Internal inhibitions and controls. In R. Hogan, J. Johnson, & S. Briggs (Eds.), *Handbook of personality psychology.* (pp. 581–614). San Diego, CA: Academic Press.

Miller, N. E. (1959). Liberalization of basic S-R concepts: Extensions to conflict behavior, motivation, and social learning. In S. Koch (Ed.), *A study of psychology as a science* (Vol. 2, pp. 196–292). New York: McGraw-Hill.

Miller, W. R., & C'deBaca, J. (1994). Quantum change: Toward a psychology of transformation. In T. Heatherton & J. Weinberger (Eds.), *Can personality change?* (pp. 253–280). Washington, DC: American Psychological Association.

Mischel, W. (1968). *Personality and assessment.* New York: Wiley.

Mongrain, M., & Emmons, R. A. (1993). *The influence of induced mood on dependency, self-criticism, ambivalence, and goal appraisals.* Unpublished manuscript, University of California, Davis.

Monte, C. F. (1999). *Beneath the mask: An introduction to theories of personality.* Fort Worth, TX: Harcourt Brace.

Murphy, G. (1947). *Personality: A biosocial approach to origins and structure.* New York: Harper & Row.

Murray, H. A. (1938). *Explorations in personality.* New York: Oxford University Press.

Murray, H. A. (1959). Preparations for the scaffold of a comprehensive system. In S. Koch (Ed.), *Psychology: A study of a science* (Vol. 3, pp. 7–54). New York: McGraw-Hill.

Murray, H. A. (1960). Two versions of man. In H. Shapley (Ed.), *Science ponders religion* (pp. 147–181). New York: Appleton-Century-Crofts.

Myers, D. G. (1978). *The human puzzle: Psychological research and Christian belief.* San Francisco: Harper & Row.

Myers, D. G. (1992). *The pursuit of happiness.* New York: William Morrow.

Myers, D. G., & Diener, E. (1995). Who is happy? *Psychological Science, 6,* 10–19.

Naguib, S. M., Geiser, P. B., & Comstock, G. W. (1968). Responses to a program of screening for cervical cancer. *Public Health Reports, 83,* 990–998.

Nasr, S. (1964). Ibn Al-'Arabi and the Sufis. In *Three Muslim sages* (pp. 83–121). Cambridge, MA: Harvard University Press.

Newberg, A. S., & d'Aquili, E. G. (1998). The neuropsychology of spiritual experience. In H. Koenig (Ed.), *Handbook of religion and mental health* (pp. 75–94). San Diego, CA: Academic Press.

Niebuhr, R. (1941). *The nature and destiny of man* (Vol. 1). New York: Scribner's.

The NIV Bible. (1984). Grand Rapids, MI: Zondervan.

Novak, M. (1996). *Business as a calling: Work and the examined life.* New York: Free Press.

Nozick, R. (1989). *The examined life.* New York: Touchstone.

Oatley, K. (1992). *Best laid schemes: The psychology of emotions.* New York: Cambridge University Press.

O'Brien, M. E. (1982). Religious faith and adjustment to long-term hemodialysis. *Journal of Religion and Health, 21,* 68–80.

Omodei, M. M., & Wearing, A. J. (1990). Need satisfaction and involvement in personal projects: Toward an integrative model of subjective well-being. *Journal of Personality and Social Psychology, 59,* 762–769.

Orias, J., Leung, L., Dosanj, S., & Sheposh, J. P. (1998, August). *Personal striving level and self-evaluation processes.* Poster presented at the annual convention of the American Psychological Association, San Francisco.

Ortony, A., Clore, G. L., & Collins, A. (1988). *The cognitive structure of emotions.* New York: Cambridge University Press.

Paloutzian, R. F. (1996). *Invitation to the psychology of religion* (2nd ed.). Needham Heights, MA: Allyn & Bacon.

Paloutzian, R. F., & Kirkpatrick, L. A. (1995). Introduction: The scope of religious influences on personal and societal well-being. *Journal of Social Issues, 51,* 1–11.

Paloutzian, R. F., Richardson, J. T., & Rambo, L. R. (in press). Religious conversion and personality change. *Journal of Personality.*

Palys, T. S., & Little, B. R. (1983). Perceived life satisfaction and the organization of personal project systems. *Journal of Personality and Social Psychology, 44,* 1221–1230.

Pargament, K. I. (1992). Of means and ends: Religion and the search for significance. *International Journal for the Psychology of Religion, 2,* 201–229.

Pargament, K. I. (1996). Religious methods of coping: Resources for the conservation and transformation of significance. In Shafranske, E. (Ed.), *Religion and the clinical practice of psychology* (pp. 215–239). Washington, DC: American Psychological Association.

Pargament, K. I. (1997). *The psychology of religion and coping: Theory, research, practice.* New York: Guilford Press.

Pargament, K. I., & Park, C. L. (1995). Merely a defense? The variety of religious means and ends. *Journal of Social Issues, 51,* 13–32.

Park, C. L., Cohen, L. H., & Murch, R. L. (1996). Assessment and prediction of stress-related growth. *Journal of Personality, 64,* 71–105.

Park, C. L., & Folkman, S. (1997). Meaning in the context of stress and coping. *Review of General Psychology, 1,* 115–144.

Parks, S. (1993). Pastoral counseling and the university. In R. J. Wicks, R. D. Parsons, & D. Capps (Eds.), *Studies in pastoral psychology, theology, and spirituality* (pp. 388–405). New York: Paulist Press.

Pavot, W., & Diener, E. (1993). Review of the Satisfaction With Life Scale. *Psychological Assessment, 5,* 164–172.

Pennebaker, J. W. (1989). Stream of consciousness and stress: Levels of thinking. In J. S. Uleman & J. A. Bargh (Eds.), *Unintended thought* (pp. 327–350). New York: Guilford Press.

Pennebaker, J. W. (1990). *Opening up: The healing power of expressing emotions.* New York: Guilford Press.

Pennebaker, J. W., Kiecolt-Glaser, J., & Glaser, R. (1989). Disclosure of traumas and immune function: Health implications for psychotherapy. *Journal of Consulting and Clinical Psychology, 56,* 239–245.

Perring, C., Oatley, K., & Smith, J. (1988). Psychiatric symptoms and conflict among personal plans. *British Journal of Medical Psychology, 61,* 167–177.

Pervin, L. A. (1983). The stasis and flow of behavior: Toward a theory of goals. In M. M. Page (Ed.), *Nebraska Symposium on Motivation* (Vol. 31, pp. 1–53). Lincoln: University of Nebraska Press.

Pervin, L. A. (1985). Personality: Current controversies, issues, directions. *Annual Review of Psychology, 36,* 83–114.

Pervin, L. A. (Ed.). (1989). *Goal concepts in personality and social psychology.* Hillsdale, NJ: Erlbaum.

Pervin, L. A. (Ed.). (1990). *Handbook of personality: Theory and research*. New York: Guilford Press.

Pervin, L. A. (1994). A critical analysis of current trait theory. *Psychological Inquiry, 5*, 103–113.

Peters, T. (1994). *Sin: Radical evil in soul and society*. Grand Rapids, MI: Eerdmans.

Piedmont, R. L. (in press). Does spirituality represent the sixth factor of personality? Spiritual transcendence and the five-factor model. *Journal of Personality*.

Pinker, S. (1997). *How the mind works*. New York: Norton.

Poloma, M. M., & Pendleton, B. F. (1990). Religious domains and general well-being. *Social Indicators Research, 22*, 255–276.

Powers, W. T. (1973). *Behavior: The control of perception*. Chicago: Aldine.

Propst, R. L. (1988). *Psychotherapy in a religious framework*. New York: Human Sciences Press.

Pruett, G. E. (1987). *The meaning and end of suffering for Freud and the Buddhist tradition*. Lanham, MD: University Press of America.

Pruyser, P. W. (1960). Some trends in the psychology of religion. *Journal of Religion, 40*, 113–129.

Ramachandran, V. S., & Blakeslee, S. (1998). *Phantoms in the brain: Probing the mysteries of the human mind*. New York: William Morrow.

Rambo, L. R. (1993). *Understanding religious conversion*. New Haven, CT: Yale University Press.

Rapkin, B. D., & Fischer, K. (1992). Personal goals of older adults: Issues in assessment and prediction. *Psychology and Aging, 7*, 127–137.

Read, S. J., & Miller, L. C. (1989). Interpersonalism: Toward a goal-based theory of persons in relationships. In L. A. Pervin (Ed.), *Goal concepts in personality and social psychology* (pp. 413–472). Hillsdale, NJ: Erlbaum.

Reid, D. (1994). *The complete book of Chinese health and healing*. Boston: Shambhala.

Reker, G. T., & Wong, P. T. P. (1988). Aging as an individual process: Toward a theory of personal meaning. In J. E. Birren & V. L. Bengston (Eds.), *Emergent theories of aging* (pp. 214–246). New York: Springer.

Richards, N. (1992). *Humility*. Philadelphia: Temple University Press.

Richards, P. S., & Bergin, A. E. (1997). *A spiritual strategy for counseling and psychotherapy*. Washington, DC: American Psychological Association.

Robbins, S. B., Lee, R. M., & Wan, T. T. (1994). Goal continuity as a mediator of early retirement adjustment. *Journal of Counseling Psychology, 41*, 18–26.

Roberts, R. C. (1991). Virtues and rules. *Philosophy and Phenomenological Research, 51*, 325–343.

Roof, W. C. (1993). *A generation of seekers: The spiritual journeys of the baby boom generation*. San Francisco: Harper.

Rook, K. S. (1984). The negative side of social interaction: Impact on psychological well-being. *Journal of Personality and Social Psychology, 46*, 1097–1108.

Rubinstein, R. L. (1994). Generativity as pragmatic spirituality. In L. E. Thomas & S. A. Eisenhandler (Eds.), *Aging and the religious dimension* (pp. 169–181). Westport, CT: Auburn House.

Ruehlman, L. S., & Wolchik, S. A. (1988). Personal goals and interpersonal support and hindrance as factors in psychological distress and well-being. *Journal of Personality and Social Psychology, 55,* 293–301.

Ryan, R. M. (1995). Psychological needs and the facilitation of integrative processes. *Journal of Personality, 63,* 397–428.

Ryan, R. M., & Frederick, C. (1997). On energy, personality, and health: Subjective vitality as a dynamic reflection of well-being. *Journal of Personality, 65,* 529–565.

Ryan, R. M., Rigby, S., & King, K. (1993). Two types of religious internalization and their relations to religious orientations and mental health. *Journal of Personality and Social Psychology, 65,* 586–596.

Ryan, R. M., Sheldon, K. M., Kasser, T., & Deci, E. L. (1996). All goals are not created equal: An organismic perspective on the nature of goals and their regulation. In P. M. Gollwitzer & J. A. Bargh (Eds.), *The psychology of action: Linking cognition and motivation to behavior* (pp. 7–26). New York: Guilford Press.

Ryff, C. D. (1989). Happiness is everything, or is it? Explorations on the meaning of psychological well-being. *Journal of Personality and Social Psychology, 57,* 1069–1081.

Ryff, C. D., & Singer, B. (1998). The contours of positive human health. *Psychological Inquiry, 9,* 1–28.

Sackeim, H. A. (1983). Self-deception, self-esteem, and depression: The adaptive value of lying to oneself. In J. Masling (Ed.), *Empirical studies of psychoanalytic theory* (Vol. 1, pp. 101–157). Hillsdale, NJ: Analytic Press.

Sacks, H. L. (1979). The effects of spiritual exercises on the integration of the self-system. *Journal for the Scientific Study of Religion, 18,* 46–50.

Salmela-Aro, K. (1992). Struggling with self: The personal projects of students seeking psychological counselling. *Scandianavian Journal of Psychology, 33,* 330–338.

Salmela-Aro, K., Nurmi, J., & Ruotsalainen, H. (1995). Personal goals of young society drop-outs. *Perceptual and Motor Skills, 80,* 1184–1186.

Salovey, P., & Sluyter, D. J. (1997). *Emotional development and emotional intelligence.* New York: Basic Books.

Santrock, J. W. (1997). *Psychology* (5th ed.). Dubuque, IA: Brown and Benchmark.

Sapolsky, R. M. (1994). *Why zebras don't get ulcers: A guide to stress, stress-related diseases, and coping.* New York: Freeman.

Saver, J. L., & Rabin, J. (1997). The neural substrates of religious experience. *Journal of Neuropsychiatry and Clinical Neurosciences, 9,* 498–510.

Sawrey, W. L., & Weisz, J. D. (1956). An experimental method of producing gastric ulcers. *Journal of Comparative and Physiological Psychology, 49,* 269–270.

Schaefer, J. A., & Moos, R. H. (1992). Life crises and personal growth. In B. N. Carpenter (Ed.), *Personal coping: Theory, research, and application* (pp. 149–170). Westport, CT: Praeger.

Scherwitz, L., & Canick, J. C. (1988). Self-reference and coronary heart disease risk. In B. K. Houston, & C. R. Snyder (Ed.), *Type A behavior pattern: Research, theory, and intervention* (pp. 146–167). New York: Wiley.

Schimmel, S. (1997). *The seven deadly sins: Jewish, Christian, and classical reflections on human psychology*. New York: Oxford University Press.

Schumaker, J. F. (Ed.). (1992). *Religion and mental health*. New York: Oxford.

Schwartzberg, S. S. (1993). Struggling for meaning: How HIV-positive gay men make sense of AIDS. *Professional Psychology: Research and Practice, 24,* 483–490.

Schwarz, N. (1990). Feelings as information: Informational and motivational functions of affective states. In E. T. Higgins & R. M. Sorrentino (Eds.), *Handbook of motivation and cognition* (Vol. 2, pp. 527–561). New York: Guilford Press.

Shafranske, E. (Ed.). (1996). *Religion and the clinical practice of psychology*. Washington, DC: American Psychological Association.

Sheldon, K. M. (1995). Creativity and goal conflict. *Creativity Research Journal, 8,* 299–306.

Sheldon, K. M., & Emmons, R. A. (1995). Comparing differentiation and integration within personal goal systems. *Personality and Individual Differences, 18,* 39–46.

Sheldon, K. M., & Kasser, T. (1995). Coherence and congruence: Two aspects of personality integration. *Journal of Personality and Social Psychology, 68,* 531–543.

Sheldon, K. M., & Kasser, T. (1998). Pursuing personal goals: Skills enable progress, but not all progress is beneficial. *Personality and Social Psychology Bulletin, 24,* 1319–1331.

Shore, E. (1997). At the center. *Parabola,* (Spring), 59–62.

Shuchter, S. R., & Zisook, S. (1993). The course of normal grief. In S. Stroebe, W. Stroebe, & R. O. Hanson (Eds.), *Handbook of bereavement: Theory, research, and intervention* (pp. 23–43). New York: Cambridge University Press.

Shulman, A. K. (1995). *Drinking the rain*. New York: Farrar, Straus & Giroux.

Silver, R. C., Boon, C., & Stones, M. H. (1983). Searching for meaning in misfortune: Making sense of incest. *Journal of Social Issues, 39,* 81–101.

Sincoff, J. B. (1990). The psychological characteristics of ambivalent people. *Clinical Psychology Review, 10,* 43–68.

Singer, J. A. (1997). *Message in a bottle: Stories of men and addiction*. New York: Free Press.

Singer, J. A., & Salovey, P. (1993). *The remembered self: Emotion and memory in personality*. New York: The Free Press.

Slife, B., Hope, C., & Nebeker, S. (1997). *Examining the relationship between religious spirituality and psychological science*. Unpublished manuscript, Brigham Young University.

Smith, C. P. (Ed.) (1992). *Motivation and personality: Handbook of thematic content analysis*. New York: Cambridge University Press.

Snarey, J. (1993). *How fathers care for the next generation: A four-decade study*. Cambridge, MA: Harvard University Press.

Spilka, B., & Bridges, R. A. (1989). Theology and psychological theory: Psychological implications of some modern theologies. *Journal of Psychology and Theology, 17,* 343–351.

Stagner, R. (1937). *Psychology of personality.* New York: McGraw-Hill.

Stein, N., Folkman, S., Trabasso, T., & Richards, A. T. (1997). Appraisal and goal processes and predictors of psychological well-being in bereaved caregivers. *Journal of Personality and Social Psychology, 72,* 872–884.

Stern, W. (1938). *General psychology from the personalist standpoint* (H. D. Spoerl, Trans.). New York: Macmillan.

Sternberg, R. J. (1990). *Metaphors of mind: Conceptions of the nature of intelligence.* New York: Cambridge University Press.

Sternberg, R. J., & Ruzgis, P. (Eds.). (1994). *Personality and intelligence.* New York: Cambridge University Press.

Stratton, G. M. (1911). *Psychology of the religious life.* London: George Allen.

Strauman, T. J., Lemieux, A. M., & Coe, C. L. (1991). Self- discrepancies and natural killer cell activity: Immunological consequences of negative self-evaluation. *Journal of Personality and Social Psychology, 65,* 165–175.

Stromberg, P. G. (1993). *Language and self–transformation: A study of the Christian conversion narrative.* New York: Cambridge University Press.

Suh, E., Diener, E., & Fujita, F. (1996). Events and subjective well-being: Only recent events matter. *Journal of Personality and Social Psychology, 70,* 1091–1102.

Taylor, R. L., & Watson, J. (1989). *They shall not hurt: Human suffering and human caring.* Boulder, CO: Colorado Associated University Press.

Taylor, S. E. (1983). Adjustment to threatening events: A theory of cognitive adaptation. *American Psychologist, 38,* 1161–1173.

Taylor, S. E., & Brown, J. D. (1988). Illusion and well-being: A social psychological perspective on mental health. *Psychological Bulletin, 103,* 193–210.

Tedeschi, R. G., & Calhoun, L. G. (1995). *Trauma and transformation.* Thousand Oaks, CA: Sage.

Tedeschi, R. G., Park, C. L., & Calhoun, L. G. (Eds). (1998). *Posttraumatic growth: Positive changes in the aftermath of crisis.* Mahwah, NJ: Erlbaum.

Tellegen, A., Lykken, D. T., Bouchard, T. J., Jr., Wilcox, K., Segal, N., & Rich, S. (1988). Personality similarity in twins reared apart and together. *Journal of Personality and Social Psychology, 54,* 1031–1039.

Templeton, J. M. (1997). *Worldwide laws of life: Two hundred eternal spiritual principles.* Radnor, PA: Templeton Press.

Tillich, P. (1948). *The shaking of the foundations.* New York: Scribner's.

Tillich, P. (1951). *Systematic theology I.* Chicago: University of Chicago Press.

Tillich, P. (1957). *Dynamics of faith.* New York: Harper & Row.

Tillich, P. (1963). *Christianity and the encounter of world religions.* New York: Columbia University Press.

Trout, D. M. (1931). *Religious behavior: An introduction to the psychological study of religion.* New York: Macmillan.

Vallacher, R. R., & Wegner, D. M. (1985). *A theory of action identification.* Hillsdale, NJ: Erlbaum.

Vande Kemp, H. (1995). Religion in college textbooks: Allport's historic 1948 report. *International Journal for the Psychology of Religion, 5,* 199–211.

Vash, C. L. (1994). *Personality and adversity: Psychospiritual aspects of rehabilitation.* New York: Springer.

Ventis, W. L. (1995). The relationships between religion and mental health. *Journal of Social Issues, 51,* 33–48.

Vergote, A. (1988). *Guilt and desire: Religious attitudes and their pathological derivatives* (M. H. Wood, Trans.). New Haven, CT: Yale University Press.

Wadsworth, M., & Ford, D. H. (1983). Assessment of personal goal hierarchies. *Journal of Counseling Psychology, 30,* 514–526.

Waller, N. G., Kojetin, B. A., Bouchard, T. J., Jr., Lykken, D. T., & Tellegen, A. (1990). Genetic and environmental influences on religious interests, attitudes, and values: A study of twins reared apart and together. *Psychological Science, 1,* 1–5.

Walters, J. M., Gardner, H. (1986). The theory of multiple intelligences: Some issues and answers. In R. J. Sternberg & R. K. Wagner (Eds.), *Practical intelligence* (pp. 163–182). New York: Cambridge University Press.

Ware, A. P., & Mendelsohn, G. A. (1997, August). *Examples and instructions: Differences in sampling idiographically assessed goals.* Poster presented at the annual meeting of the American Psychological Association, Chicago.

Waterman, A. S. (1993). Finding something to do or someone to be: A eudaimonist perspective on identity formation. In J. Kroger (Ed.), *Discussions on ego identity* (pp. 147–167). Hillsdale, NJ: Erlbaum.

Watson, D., & Tellegen, A. (1985). Toward a consensual structure of mood. *Psychological Bulletin, 98,* 219–245.

Watts, F., & Williams, M. (1988). *The psychology of religious knowing.* New York: Cambridge University Press.

Weinberger, D. A. (1990). The construct validity of the repressive coping style. In J. Singer (Ed.), *Repression and dissociation: Implications for personality theory, psycopathology, and health* (pp. 337–386). Chicago: University of Chicago Press.

Weiner, B. (1986). Attribution, emotion, and action. In R. M. Sorrentino & E. T. Higgins (Eds.), *Handbook of motivation and cognition* (pp. 281–312). New York: Guilford Press.

Weiss, H. M., & Knight, P. A. (1980). The utility of humility: Self-esteem, information search, and problem-solving efficiency. *Organizational Behavior and Human Decision Processes, 25,* 216–223.

Werner, H., & Kaplan, B. (1956). The developmental approach to cognition: Its relevance to the psychological interpretation of anthropological and ethno-linguistic data. *American Anthropologist, 58,* 866–880.

Westen, D. (1992). The cognitive self and the psychoanalytic self: Can we put our selves together? *Psychological Inquiry, 3,* 1–13.

Wiggins, J. S. (Ed.). (1996). *The five-factor model of personality: Theoretical perspectives.* New York: Guilford Press.

Wilensky, R. (1983). *Planning and understanding: A computational approach to human reasoning.* Reading, MA: Addison-Wesley.

Wilson, E. O. (1978). *On human nature.* Cambridge, MA: Harvard University Press.

Wilson, M. R. (1989). *Our father Abraham: Jewish roots of the Christian faith.* Grand Rapids, MI: Eerdmans.

Winter, D. G., John, O. P., Stewart, A. J., Klohnen, E. C., & Duncan, L. E. (1998). Traits and motives: Toward an integration of two traditions in personality research. *Psychological Review, 105,* 230–250.

Wong, P. T. P. (1998). Meaning-centered counseling. In P. T. P. Wong & P. S. Fry (Eds.), *The human quest for meaning* (pp. 395–435). Mahwah, NJ: Erlbaum.

Wong, P. T. P., & Fry, P. S. (Eds.). (1998). *The human quest for meaning: A handbook of psychological research and clinical applications.* Mahwah, NJ: Erlbaum.

Worthington, E. L., Kurusu, T. A., McCullough, M., & Sandage, S. J. (1996). Empirical research on religion and psychotherapeutic processes and outcomes: A 10-year review and research prospectus. *Psychological Bulletin, 119,* 448–487.

Wulff, D. M. (1997). *Psychology of religion: Classic and contemporary* (2nd ed.). New York: Wiley.

Wuthnow, R. (1998). *After heaven: Spirituality in America since the 1950's.* Berkeley, CA: University of California Press.

Yalom, I. (1980). *Existential psychotherapy.* New York: Basic Books.

Yetim, U. (1993). Life satisfaction: A study based on the organization of personal projects. *Social Indicators Research, 29,* 277–289.

Yinger, J. M. (1967). Pluralism, religion, and secularism. *Journal for the Scientific Study of Religion, 6,* 17–28.

Zagzebski, L. T. (1996). *Virtues of the mind.* New York: Cambridge University Press.

Zautra, A. J., Potter, P. T., & Reich, J. W. (1998). The independence of affects is context-dependent: An integrative model of the relationship between positive and negative affect. In K. W. Schaie & M. P. Lawton (Eds.), *Annual review of gerontology and geriatrics* (Vol. 17, pp. 75–103). New York: Springer.

Zeldow, P. B., Daugherty, S. R., & McAdams, D. P. (1988). Intimacy, power, and psychological health. *Journal of Nervous and Mental Disease, 176,* 172–187.

Zinnbauer, B. J., & Pargament, K. I. (1998). Spiritual conversion: A study of religious change among college students. *Journal for the Scientific Study of Religion, 37,* 161–180.

Index